Maximum Energy for Life

A 21-Day Strategic Plan to Feel
Great, Reverse the Aging Process,
and Optimize Your Health

Mackie Shilstone

John Wiley & Sons, Inc.

Copyright © 2003 by Mackie Shilstone. All rights reserved

Published by John Wiley & Sons, Inc., Hoboken, New Jersey
Published simultaneously in Canada

The "Performance Assessment Questionnaire" and "How Do I Approach Goal Setting?" are used by permission of F. Dean Sunseri, L.P.C., Life Coach, The Evergreen Wellness Center; "How Vulnerable Are You to Stress" is used by permission of The University of California at Berkeley Wellness Letter, © 1995; the material under the heading "Biofeedback: Feel the Difference between Arousal and Relaxation" and the eight meditative exercises are from The High Performance Mind: Mastering Brainwaves for Insight, Healing, and Creativity (Jeremy P. Tarcher/Putnam) and is used by permission of the author, Anna Wise © 1995; the material on Attitude Breathing is copyrighted by the Institute of HeartMath and is used by permission; the "At-Home Body Fat Test for Males" and the "At-Home Body Fat Test for Females" are from the book Turn Up the Heat: Unlock the Fat-Burning Power of Your Metabolism (Viking) and are used by permission of the author, Philip L. Goglia © 2002; "Top Twenty Carbohydrates Ingested by Americans" and "Acceptable (Low) Glycemic Foods" are used by permission of the Glycemic Research Institute, Washington, D.C.; the "Questionnaire for Nutritional Assessment" and the material under the heading "Eat Healthy with These Nutritional Guidelines" are used by permission of E. C. Henley, Ph.D., R.D. © 2002; some of the material in "The "Wellness Organizer" was adapted from the "Skinny Box" developed by Hal C. Becker, Ph.D., and is used by his permission; the questionnaire PAR-Q AND YOU is reprinted from the 1994 revised version of the Physical Activity Readiness Questionnaire (PAR-Q AND YOU). PAR-Q AND YOU is a copyrighted, pre-exercise screen owned by the Canadian Society for Exercise Physiology; "A Ten-Year Risk Evaluation for Men and Women" in the appendix was published by NIH (the National Institutes of Health), Publication No. 01-3305, May 2001.

No part of this publication may be reproduced, stored in a retrieval system, or transmitted in any form or by any means, electronic, mechanical, photocopying, recording, scanning, or otherwise, except as permitted under Section 107 or 108 of the 1976 United States Copyright Act, without either the prior written permission of the Publisher, or authorization through payment of the appropriate per-copy fee to the Copyright Clearance Center, 222 Rosewood Drive, Danvers, MA 01923, (978) 750-8400, fax (978) 750-4470. Requests to the Publisher for permission should be addressed to the Permissions Department, John Wiley & Sons, Inc., 111 River Street, Hoboken, NJ 07030, (201) 748-6011, fax (201) 748-6008, email: permcoordinator@wiley.com.

Limit of Liability/Disclaimer of Warranty: While the publisher and the author have used their best efforts in preparing this book, they make no representations or warranties with respect to the accuracy or completeness of the contents of this book and specifically disclaim any implied warranties of merchantability or fitness for a particular purpose. No warranty may be created or extended by sales representatives or written sales materials. The advice and strategies contained herein may not be suitable for your situation. You should consult with a professional where appropriate. Neither the publisher nor the author shall be liable for any loss of profit or any other commercial damages, including but not limited to special, incidental, consequential, or other damages.

For general information about our other products and services, please contact our Customer Care Department within the United States at (800) 762-2974, outside the United States at (317) 572-3993 or fax (317) 572-4002.

Wiley also publishes its books in a variety of electronic formats. Some content that appears in print may not be available in electronic books. For more information about Wiley products, visit our web site at www.wiley.com.

Library of Congress Cataloging-in-Publication Data

Shilstone, Mackie.
    Maximum energy for life : a 21-day strategic plan to feel great,
  reverse the aging process, and optimize your health / Mackie Shilstone.
        p. cm.
    Includes bibliographical references and index.
        ISBN 0-471-23537-7 (Cloth)
    1. Health.   2. Physical fitness.   I. Title.
        RA776 .S53723 2003
        613—dc21   2002014019

Printed in the United States of America

10 9 8 7 6 5 4 3 2 1

This book is dedicated to my loving family—
my wife, Sandy, my two sons, Scott and Spencer,
my mother, Frances—and to the spirit in the heart
of the strongest and bravest man I've ever known
in my life, my father, Cecil.

Contents

Foreword

by Steve Wynn

I first met Mackie Shilstone back in 1993, although I'd been aware of his reputation in the sports performance field for many years. Mackie's revolutionary performance enhancement strategies came to my attention in 1985 when he made history by training Michael Spinks to be the first light heavyweight boxer to move up and take the title from the heavyweight champion of the world, Larry Holmes.

Because Las Vegas, where I lived, worked, and owned several properties, was where many important boxing matches took place, Mackie and the athletes he worked with were there often. In 1993 Evander Holyfield was the champion and Riddick Bowe was preparing to challenge his title. Holyfield was considered to be one of the most conditioned athletes in the world, so it was going to be quite a contest.

I was curious to see how Mackie's innovative techniques worked up close, so during the last weeks of Bowe's training I invited him and Bowe to do one of their cardiovascular training runs at Shadow Creek, my private golf course. I noticed that Mackie had Bowe wear a heart monitor, a training technique I'd never seen before. When I remarked about it, he said that he was maneuvering Bowe's heart rate up and down to simulate what he would actually experience during the fight.

I asked Mackie if I could work with him a bit during his off hours, and he kindly consented. He also utilized a heart-rate monitor on me, and it was the first time I had ever understood how managing your heart rate could affect your performance. As a busy entrepreneur and developer, stress was something I was accustomed to. One of Mackie's specialties was performance stress management, and we had some enlightening conversations about it. He explained to me that boxing was largely learning how to utilize applied stress, the stress of repeatedly inflicting blows upon your opponent and the stress you experience trying to get out of the way of your opponent's punches. I immediately saw the ramifications of his philosophy for my own work.

He also taught me dynamic core stabilization techniques for my body, using gymnastic balls. Every workout facility has those now, but back in 1993, this technique was revolutionary. I soon realized that Mackie's training techniques were ten years ahead of everyone else's. They still are today.

Eight years later, in 2001, I had just sold many of my properties and felt that I needed to invest some serious time in improving my health. Even though I could travel anywhere in the world and work with anyone to help me develop a program for fitness and performance management, I felt that the person who truly could serve me the best was Mackie Shilstone. Three weeks later my wife, Elaine, and I were in New Orleans where Mackie works and lives.

The first thing Mackie did was to put us through the battery of innovative medical diagnostic tests he used at his Center for Performance Enhancement and Lifestyle Management. I was deeply impressed with his ability to utilize leading edge medical procedures and apply the information they gave him to perfecting human performance. My wife and I were given tests for cardiovascular fitness, a general medical screening, and some tests I'd never heard of before, such as screening for cardiovascular risk factors such as lipoprotein (a), c-reactive protein, and homocysteine levels. All of the latter tests had been available for some time, but not many people knew how to integrate them into the creation of a plan for optimum health and performance. This is what Mackie does best.

I learned many things about myself during that visit. The first thing I discovered was that I was training way too hard. As someone who has developed many properties and is currently working on a major development in the Las Vegas area, I've always known that you have to push hard to succeed. But Mackie's program taught me many valuable tools about how to recover from hard work, and how to create periods of downtime in my exercise program so that my muscles could rebuild and recover for maximum results. My energy increased, and my body fat went down. During the course of my workday, I no longer had to work as hard internally to manage stress and fatigue. I was experiencing the same level of work and stress, but the improvements in my overall health and the stress management techniques Mackie taught me showed me how to handle it much more effectively. I could tolerate work pressures better and pay less of a price to do it, since I could now recover so much quicker.

No matter how successful you are, the one thing you can't buy is your health. But as I did, you can put the expertise and cutting edge knowledge of Mackie Shilstone to work for you. This book represents a strategic management plan for anyone who is concerned about where he or she is in relation to his or her health and fitness levels. It is also the ultimate book for helping you to identify where you want to go and how best to achieve your performance goals. The performance management plan he offers in this book is truly a road map to success that you will want to use for the rest of your life.

Mackie is a man of true vision, someone who knows how to put his knowledge into a form that is both understandable and easy to assimilate. Because he so thoroughly enjoys what he does, his enthusiasm and energy are always high. No one I have ever met has more of an ability to motivate others not only to feel good about themselves but also to get the most they can out of their performance, every step of the way.

Acknowledgments

I would like to thank the following people for their invaluable help with this book:

My loving wife, Sandy, and my sons, Scott and Spencer, for their patience and understanding to help me fulfill this dream.

My friend and collaborator, Joy Parker. During the years that we have worked together, Joy has been able to get into my mind and clearly capture my voice, expressing my ideas in a way that is truly remarkable. She has the ability to take extremely complex issues and write about them in a way that is appealing and understandable. This book represents the culmination of twenty-five years of my work, and I would never have entrusted it to anyone else.

My literary agent, Bonnie Solow, for taking my dream, helping me to bring it to fruition, and then taking it out into the world and finding a home for it.

Tom Miller, who bought into my energy and passion for this work. His skillful editing and dedication to the highest standards of excellence have turned this into a book that will hopefully help thousands of people to reach their health and performance goals.

Carl "Chip" Lavie, M.D., for his invaluable input on heart disease and health.

Mike Derrington of Protein Technologies for supporting the book and helping to bring some valuable consultants to the table during its writing.

Dean Sunseri, for the important evaluation questionnaires he designed for my readers.

E.C. Henley, for her nutritional program and questionnaire.

Molly Kimball, for designing the food programs.

My assistant Kim Cummings, for her invaluable help in coordinating several important phases of this project, and for her loyalty and friendship.

Judy Johnson for taking the photographs of the Pro Circuit.

Ken Kachtik, general manager, and my fellow employees at Elmwood Fitness Center for letting me be a part of their team.

The physicians, nurses, and staff at the Ochsner Clinic Foundation, for their continued support.

Jim Flarity, for his help with the "rate of perceived exertion."

And to all of my clients who have so generously given their time and shared their stories with me. You have all made this book so much more meaningful, and I thank you for your dedication to your health and performance. You are the true champions.

To my PEP team, for their undying support and loyalty.

To my friend Mark Letendre, for his insight and support.

Introduction

When I was a young man, my goal was to be a walk-on wide receiver for a major college football team. My size was against me, though. At five feet eight inches and 140 pounds, I was the smallest guy at the Tulane University tryouts. Yet I persevered, creating a strategic plan of rigorous exercise and nutrition and developing an attitude that said, "Never give up." I ended up being the smallest guy on the team and the smallest player in the country, but I earned my varsity letter.

This experience became the template for my life. First, you have to evaluate and understand your capabilities. From there you have to learn how to downplay the negatives and focus on the positives. Then you have to learn how to nurture your passion so that the distractions and setbacks you encounter along the way do not defeat you. This book will show you how.

The most demanding, high-profile arena for achievement—the place where peak performance most often equals success—is the world of professional sports. As someone who has motivated more than a thousand athletes to break records; to win Super Bowls, World Series, and heavyweight championships; and even to come back from cancer, addictions, and traumatic injury, I know how to help you set performance goals and achieve optimum health and fitness.

For more than twenty-five years, I have built a career helping world-class athletes to be faster, more focused, healthier, and live more balanced lifestyles. I have helped them reach new levels of peak performance and achieve even greater success at what they do best. When Michael Spinks made history by becoming the *first* light-heavyweight boxer to successfully win the world heavyweight boxing title against Larry Holmes, he had my program behind him. When basketball great Marcus Camby of the New York Knicks wanted to revitalize his career, he turned to me for help. When all-star Ozzie Smith at the age of thirty wanted just three more years on the baseball diamond with the Saint Louis Cardinals, he put his performance coaching into my hands. His career continued another eleven years

1

until he retired at the age of forty-one. Three months after baseball star Brett Butler had surgery and radiation treatment for cancer, he put in seventeen days of rigorous training with me and made a miraculous comeback with the Dodgers, scoring the winning run in the game against the Pittsburgh Pirates. I have devised performance longevity programs for professional athletes that have extended their careers far beyond what is normally expected. For example, in the body-destroying NFL, where the average career expectancy is only three and a half years, I enabled Lomas Brown to play for more than sixteen years.

Behind the scenes of the most competitive arenas on Earth, I have tested and mastered physical, emotional, mental, and health strategies and principles that can mean the difference between failure and success, between giving up or breaking through to the next level of achievement.

My work hasn't only been with professional athletes and celebrities. My passion for promoting top performance and career longevity has led to the development of the Mackie Shilstone Center for Performance Enhancement and Lifestyle Management at the Elmwood Fitness Center in New Orleans. I have taken what I learned working with champion athletes and distilled it into a program of preventative health, weight loss through proper nutrition, exercise, and stress management that has helped thousands of everyday men and women achieve optimum performance in their careers and the level of emotional balance they long for in their personal lives. To me there are no distinctions between professional athletes and the average person, only different target goals and differing training times to reach those goals.

Now, for the first time, I have distilled my twenty-five years of insights and secrets about health, nutrition, stress management, and performance longevity into a book for the ordinary reader seeking ways to improve performance and commitment to excellence in any arena of his or her life.

Over the last decade, I have become increasingly alarmed at the worsening state of health in North America. Even though we are the wealthiest society on the face of the earth with the most advanced system of medical care, we are becoming sicker, year by year.

The fault does not lie with some mysterious Factor X that has invaded our bodies, but with our loss of control over our lifestyles.

Back in 1905, only 5 percent of the population was obese. That figure has soared. The long hours we work, the enormous stress that is part of modern life, the reduced time we have to spend with our families, the processed foods that make up most of our diets, and our lack of planned exercise and physical activity have all contributed to an epidemic rise in disease processes such as cardiovascular illness and type 2 diabetes. Even though the bookstore shelves are filled with descriptions of the latest fads in exercise, dieting, or self-motivation, these programs clearly aren't getting the job done. By all accounts, we North Americans should be a lot healthier than we are.

To really comprehend the truth of our predicament, consider the prevalence of *preventable* diseases in our culture. All of the health problems listed below are killing us in greater numbers every year. Yet all of them can be avoided, improved, or completely cured by proper nutrition, exercise, stress management, and other lifestyle changes.

- Currently, 59.4 percent of adults in the United States over the age of twenty—approximately 97 million people—are overweight or obese, and this figure has increased by 8 percent in the last ten years. Being overweight or obese can increase your risk of life-threatening health conditions such as heart disease, some types of cancer, stroke, diabetes, and arteroschlerosis. Losing weight automatically decreases your risk for these diseases.
- An article in the *New York Times* reported that between 1990 and 1998 there was a 33 percent increase in cases of type 2 diabetes. An alarming 70 percent of these new cases are individuals in their thirties. Doctors estimate that more than five million people in the United States have diabetes *without knowing it,* since the disease produces few or no symptoms in its early stages. Doctors attribute much of this rise to lack of exercise and the prevalence of being overweight.
- The American Medical Association states that 11.9 percent of those living in the United States suffer from severe fatigue. Of this number, only 2.2 percent have symptoms of fatigue that cannot be attributed to physical causes. That means that nearly one out of ten people experience chronic or debilitating exhaustion that is rooted in physiological causes that are completely avoidable.

- According to Dr. James M. Rippe in his book *The Joint Prescription,* an estimated 50 percent of all people over the age of thirty have a problem with at least one joint. A number of studies conducted over the last few decades clearly show that joint problems contribute to the development of other diseases such as heart disease, diabetes, further joint problems, and a poorer quality of life. Many joint problems are caused or exacerbated by incorrect exercise or by the lack of exercise.
- Long-term stress can either kill you or greatly decrease the quality of your life and health. Stress leads to hormonal imbalance, weight gain, low energy, depressed immune function, decreased physical and mental health, job burnout, loss of productivity and creativity, and many diseases such as cancer, heart disease, and lung ailments. No one can avoid having a certain amount of stress in his or her life, but there are many effective ways to manage it. I will show you how.
- Most people believe that sarcopenia, a loss of muscle mass, and bone loss are the inevitable results of aging. But lack of physical activity and improper nutrition are what really cause these conditions.
- Heart disease is the number one killer in North America. Yet according to doctors, heart disease could be almost completely eradicated in people under age sixty-five if they exercised regularly, ate nutritious foods, and managed their stress.

This Book Could Save Your Life

So what can you do about all of this? First, you must be willing to take control of your health. You might be walking around with a serious health condition and not even know it. For example, consider that of the 1.5 million people who have heart attacks every year, 60 percent had no warning symptoms before the first attack. There are 18 million people diagnosed with diabetes in the United States, but doctors have estimated that another 5 million don't even know they have this condition because they feel no symptoms until the disease has progressed.

A lot of us are so used to living with pain, levels of exhaustion, lack of joy in our lives, and daily stress that we aren't even aware of feeling bad anymore. Ask yourself honestly, when was the last time you didn't feel some kind of daily pain in your body? Pain is a signal that something is wrong. How many mornings do you wake up feeling tired? Consistent lack of energy is a signal that something isn't working right in your body.

Most people do not realize that to a large extent, we can control not only how long we live but also the overall quality of our lives for years to come. People used to believe that the factors that influenced our health were divided fifty-fifty between our heredity and our environment. I'm here to tell you that the percentages are more like 33 percent heredity and 66 percent environment.

Which means that we all have a great deal more control over our health and our performance levels than we think we do. Isn't it time that you sat down and took the time to give yourself a real evaluation of your physical health, your risk factors for disease, your emotional well-being, and your levels of stress?

What This Book Can Do for You

There are few books on the market today that can help you to thoroughly evaluate where you are emotionally and physically. This book is designed not only to enable you to understand clearly where you are at this point in time, but also to provide you with a strategic performance management plan to enhance the overall quality of your life. Here are some of the benefits you will get from reading this book:

1. For the first time in your life, you will understand why health is your greatest asset. Health is the area in your life that you have the most control over and in which you can effect the greatest change. If you increase your level of health, you automatically increase your performance. If you increase your performance levels, you will improve all aspects of your life: your career opportunities, your passion for living, your energy levels, and the quality of your personal relationships. When your emotional and physical health improve, everything improves.
2. This book clearly shows you what your health risks are *before* they become a serious problem and how to self-diagnose the critical disease factors that can take you out.
3. It will show you how to decrease and manage your stress levels effectively to improve the quality of your life.

4. Following the program in this book will enable you to not only live longer, but also to have an outstanding quality of life no matter how old you are.

5. This book will teach you how to identify your energy style and to learn how to best work with it. All of us are born with only so much energy. The secret to not running out is learning how to work effectively *with* your own personal style and not *against* it.

6. This book offers a state-of-the-art nutritional plan to increase performance, promote weight loss, and enhance youthful longevity. This plan has worked for thousands of athletes and ordinary men and women.

7. This book describes my Pro Circuit Exercise Program, a unique workout that has helped thousands of athletes and ordinary people achieve both strength training and aerobic conditioning within one forty-five-minute workout done three times a week.

Why This Book Is Unique

I believe that this book offers readers benefits that other books can't match for a number of reasons.

First, it reflects the passion and dedication I bring to my work. There is nothing in life that gives me more joy and satisfaction than helping men and women achieve their performance goals, whether they are world-class athletes, CEOs, members of the police force, lawyers, politicians, working fathers and mothers, performing artists, business people, or up-and-coming high school and college athletes who are aiming for the pros.

Second, few authors are able to bring to the table a track record like mine. I have not only dedicated my life to studying the principles I describe in this book, but also I live them every single day. I am fifty-one, yet I have the health and performance age of a man of nineteen. I teach my health management system in a number of academic venues and have appointments at the School of Public Health and Preventative Medicine at the Louisiana State University Health Sciences Center, at Nichols State University in the Allied Health Division of Sports Medicine, and at the Tulane University with the A.B. Freeman School of Business Studies. Recently I was asked to join the board of directors of the National Mental Health Association in

Washington, D.C. Only thirty-one individuals in the entire United States have been so honored. I am also the Special Adviser in the Sports Nutrition Section of the U. S. Olympic Committee.

How the Book Is Set Up

This book is an exact duplicate of how I run my performance enhancement programs with my professional athletes and my business athletes, the men and women who venture daily into the business arena. Reading it is like hiring me and my staff of elite advisers to take you step by step through all of the physical and emotional health evaluations, that will be used to design a customized nutrition program for you and to help you create the ideal exercise program, tailored for your personal schedule and needs. Along the way, you will have the benefit of drawing upon feedback and coaching from the team of experts that I work with daily: top-of-the-line doctors and cardiologists, nutritionists, and a skilled psychologist.

In the first part of this book, you will learn how to examine your overall performance on a number of levels. I will give you tools and questionnaires that will enable you to discover your energy style, manage your fear, successfully set and achieve goals, and reduce stress. This section will help you to understand how stress works in the body, how to evaluate your stress levels, and how to apply leading edge stress management techniques I have learned from many experts and used for decades in my life and when coaching my clients.

Next, with the help of the skilled doctors with whom I work at my Center for Performance Enhancement and Lifestyle Management at the Elmwood Fitness Center, a division of the Ochsner Clinic Foundation, I will walk you through a thorough health self-evaluation. Together we will look at risk factors such as the Body Mass Index and waist measurement, and see how many major diseases such as cardiovascular illness and diabetes can be improved or completely avoided as you get older through easy-to-follow lifestyle modifications. I place special emphasis on heart health, since heart disease is the most prevalent disease in our society and the one most easily cured.

Since nutrition is one of the foundation stones of great health, two skilled nutritionists and I will take you on a tour of how foods work, the prevalent myths about diet and weight loss, what good nutrition consists of, and some fourteen-day programs featuring delicious menus.

Now you are ready for the Mackie Shilstone Pro Circuit Exercise Program. I know of no other program that enables you to combine the benefits of a balanced strength training program with core stabilization and cardiovascular training in a single workout. My clients have experienced tremendous benefits from this program, including loss of pounds, loss of inches, increased cardiovascular capacity (including a lower resting heart rate), greater muscular strength, greater bone density, and a lower percentage of body fat to lean muscle. My Pro Circuit workout has become the preferred exercise program for major league baseball umpires, and it is currently the official training program for the more than 1,700 members of the New Orleans Police Department.

Then I will show you how to renew your passion and motivation for your career and personal life.

Finally, I have designed a twenty-one-day program for you that includes all of these elements. These easy-to-follow guidelines will expertly shepherd you through my performance enhancement program just as if I were right there in the room with you.

This book represents the legacy of my twenty-five years of performance enhancement training. It embraces both the science and the passion that I bring to my work with my clients. I know that it will help you improve the quality of your life, health, and performance as well as increase your joy of living more than you ever dreamed possible. It is my personal pleasure to share my secrets and strategies with you right now. Let's begin.

PART ONE

Secrets and Strategies to Manage Your Energy and Reduce Your Stress

1

Discover the Art of Maximum Performance

Are You a Prospect or a Suspect?

In sports, a talented player who is just starting out in the game is known as a "prospect," someone who is on the verge of accomplishing great things for his team. But if he doesn't live up to his promise on the playing field, he soon becomes "suspect," a person who is failing to live up to his potential. When this happens, his performance must improve or he is off the team.

I watched this happen with J.J. McCleskey when he was a seven-year veteran with the Arizona Cardinals. When the tremendously talented J.J. was unable to complete the season four years in a row due to nagging injuries, he became suspect. His coach told him, "I don't know what you're doing in the off-season to get ready for the game, but whatever it is, you need to change it or you will have to start looking for another team." I discovered that J.J.'s problem was repetitive hamstring pulls due to overstriding and improper training practices. After working with me during the off-season, J.J. was able to play the entire sixteen-game season. In fact, he was better in the last four games than most guys were in the first games of the season, and he ended up being a Pro Bowl alternate that year.

We all start out in life as a prospect, with a balanced physical, emotional, and mental system. As we age, however, our experiences tend to throw us off balance to varying degrees if we don't learn to compensate. As the stresses of life and work add up, our health and stamina tend to decrease and we begin to lose the focus necessary for maximum performance levels. Even when we have tremendous experience and knowledge, we can still become suspect.

The following Performance Assessment Questionnaire serves as a tool to help you evaluate where you are now. Read each statement and check "never," "sometimes," or "always," depending on how accurately the statement matches your current lifestyle performance levels. The eventual goal is to check off "always" for most questions. The areas where you check "never" or "sometimes" are the ones that need attention. Make a note of these areas and use the tools I offer in this book to improve them.

Performance Assessment Questionnaire

Psychological, Emotional, and Spiritual Performance

	Never	Some-times	Always
1. I spend at least fifteen minutes a day in meditation.	☐	☐	☐
2. I am able to manage all my emotions well.	☐	☐	☐
3. I have no addictions or self-destructive compulsive behaviors.	☐	☐	☐
4. I have an intuitive sense of my purpose and I am living it now.	☐	☐	☐
5. I have a close friend to whom I talk on an emotional level.	☐	☐	☐
6. I am someone who is willing to constantly increase my knowledge.	☐	☐	☐
7. My actions are in alignment with my personal standards.	☐	☐	☐
8. I invest time, money, and energy in improving my spiritual and emotional well-being.	☐	☐	☐
9. I regularly have time for my hobbies and fun activities.	☐	☐	☐
10. I laugh a lot.	☐	☐	☐

Environmental Performance

11. My home is a place of relaxation and safety.	☐	☐	☐
12. My career environment is healthy and life giving.	☐	☐	☐

	Never	Some-times	Always

13. I am comfortable and happy in the neighborhood where I live. ☐ ☐ ☐
14. My home has lots of natural light and plants. ☐ ☐ ☐
15. My bedroom allows me to sleep comfortably. ☐ ☐ ☐
16. The air quality of my home and work environment is good. ☐ ☐ ☐
17. My papers and files are neatly organized. ☐ ☐ ☐
18. I consistently get rid of anything that I have not used in a year (e.g., clothes, tools, books, and furniture). ☐ ☐ ☐
19. All my electronic equipment works well and does not need repair. ☐ ☐ ☐
20. My home and work environments are neat and clean. ☐ ☐ ☐

Physical Performance

21. I consistently fuel my body with healthful foods and drink purified water. ☐ ☐ ☐
22. I exercise regularly. ☐ ☐ ☐
23. I am treating all my physical problems. ☐ ☐ ☐
24. I have yearly physicals. ☐ ☐ ☐
25. I take vitamin supplements daily. ☐ ☐ ☐
26. My alcohol and/or sugar intake is minimal. ☐ ☐ ☐
27. I get enough sleep on a regular basis. ☐ ☐ ☐
28. I rarely need to function on adrenaline. ☐ ☐ ☐
29. I have many healthy ways to help me relax and rejuvenate. ☐ ☐ ☐
30. I am content with my present weight. ☐ ☐ ☐

Relationship Performance

31. I have no unfinished business in any of my past relationships. ☐ ☐ ☐
32. I set good boundaries with people who drain my energy. ☐ ☐ ☐
33. I spend more than enough quality time with my family. ☐ ☐ ☐
34. I have surrounded myself with a community that gives me a sense of love and belonging. ☐ ☐ ☐

	Never	Some-times	Always
35. I have a mentor.	☐	☐	☐
36. I communicate my needs and desires honestly and directly.	☐	☐	☐
37. I do not talk about other people in a negative manner.	☐	☐	☐
38. I am very respectful of the people in my life.	☐	☐	☐
39. I have a good balance between nurturing my relationships and completing my tasks, jobs, and responsibilities.	☐	☐	☐
40. When I realize that I have harmed someone, I easily admit my mistake and apologize sincerely.	☐	☐	☐

Financial Performance

	Never	Some-times	Always
41. My financial assets to financial debt ratio is at least 2:1.	☐	☐	☐
42. My taxes are up-to-date.	☐	☐	☐
43. I have a completed will that is accurate and updated.	☐	☐	☐
44. I save 10 percent of my income.	☐	☐	☐
45. I pay my bills in a timely manner.	☐	☐	☐
46. My credit cards are paid out each month.	☐	☐	☐
47. I am well insured.	☐	☐	☐
48. I live within my present income and not on future expectations.	☐	☐	☐
49. I have six months of living expenses saved in a bank account.	☐	☐	☐
50. I have a written financial plan for the next year.	☐	☐	☐

Add up the number of responses in each category and fill in the blanks below.

Peak Performance (Always)___
Improvement Needed (Sometimes, Never)___

As you work your way through this book, you can come back to this questionnaire again and again to reassess your progress.

2

Seven Secrets to Put You at the Top of Your Form

There is a saying in the field of boxing: "It is easier to win the heavy-weight championship than to keep it." It is not enough merely to achieve the position you have always wanted. Remaining successful means continuing to be a good prospect—showing your colleagues, your employees, your boss, your coworkers, and your rivals that you are someone who continues to perform at the height of his or her powers, someone who is always on the edge of new accomplishments. A good prospect projects confidence, energy, and inspiration. He or she knows how to pull off the difficult coup, to land the big client, and sometimes even to surpass others' expectations.

How do you remain a prospect over the length of your career? The secret is to understand this: performance doesn't just happen. It must be managed like an asset.

To continue to be an outstanding player, you need to develop strategies for bringing your body, mind, and emotions back into balance. You need to evaluate your health and make intelligent choices about nutrition, exercise, stress management, and lifestyle. You need to get clear about what you really want out of your job and your significant relationships. Once you know that, you can set goals and take specific steps toward achieving them.

In my twenty-five years of working with world-class athletes and high-powered men and women, I have come up with seven strategies to keep you at the top of your form.

Secret 1: Reduce Your Health Age to Increase Your Performance Levels

All of us have a chronological age and a health age. One of the hardest tasks we face in the workplace and in life is learning how to manage our health and performance so that the wear and tear of the job doesn't make us old before our time.

We have all seen men and women who slow down and become old before their time, with a health age much greater than their chronological age. The person who burns the candle at both ends might be fifty but looks and feels like he's seventy.

On the other hand, we all know incredibly youthful and energetic individuals who might be fifty, but look, feel, and perform like a thirty-year-old. Their health age—their general level of fitness—is below their chronological age. The factors that determine our health age include body fat percentage, resting heart rate, upper body and lower back strength, metabolic rate (normal thyroid), cholesterol, fasting glucose, and triglyceride levels. Those in our society who have a lower health age are the new elite because they have the energy to perform dynamically while others are struggling to maintain the status quo. For example, I have one sixty-seven-year-old client, Alvin Edinburgh, who is so fit he was chosen to be one of the Olympic torchbearers.

When I turned fifty, my doctor told me I had the health age of a nineteen-year-old. This is not just luck or good genes. It has everything to do with how you manage your greatest asset, your health. Achieving and maintaining optimum health in your thirties, forties, and fifties are governed by very specific lifestyle choices—as are maintaining physical vitality, a good mental outlook, and passion during your last decades of life. The best news is that it is never too late to start.

Doctors used to say that our health was 50 percent heredity and 50 percent environment. They have since revised those percentages to 33 percent heredity and 66 percent environment. So aside from serious injuries or inherited health problems, you have a tremendous amount of control over your health age and, therefore, your performance age.

Poor Health Dulls Your Performance Edge

Sometimes disease or ill heath can cause you to lose your performance edge. Recently, Louis Congemi, mayor of the city of Kenner,
Louisiana, came to me for help. In childhood this man had con-
tracted mitochondrial myopathy, a rare disease that causes difficulty
in the extraction of nutrients from food, resulting in muscle atrophy.
The mitrochondria are the power packs in the cells that are responsible for energy production. This is the same disease from which
American bicyclist Greg LeMond, three-time winner of the Tour de
France, suffered. LeMond's condition forced him to retire in 1994.

Mayor Congemi was usually able to keep the effects of this disease process under control, but he felt that he wanted to do more to
improve his exercise capability. When the doctor he consulted
needed assistance, Mayor Congemi sought me out because he knew
my reputation for finding solutions for people with serious health
problems. He'd heard of the work I'd done helping Brett Butler to
recover from cancer, and he knew that I had assisted in the design of
the highly successful Pro Circuit program for the Kenner Police
Department. Based on the results he had seen among the police officers, he believed that I could help him to find a health and nutritional regimen that would at least improve his condition. If not, he
knew he would face a tougher challenge as he became older.

Since the mayor had a rare illness, we found ourselves largely in
uncharted territory. Most doctors, including the one the mayor had
consulted, seemed to know little or nothing about his condition. My
physiologist, Dr. Flaherty, and I researched everything we could find
on the disease and came up with a three-point program to counteract
its effects and rebuild the muscle tissue the mayor had lost. First, we
worked to increase his immune system so that his symptoms would
lessen and he would have the physical stamina to better resist the
degenerative effects of his illness. Second, we created a special exercise program for him that would rebuild his strength and increase his
lean muscle mass. This involved designing a workout routine for him
that would allow him consistent improvement without exhausting
him. To do so, we gave him every advantage we could think of. We
warmed up his muscles in the sauna prior to exercise and identified
his fatigue point so we would never overtire him during his workout.
Lastly, to support his workout and help him gain weight, we prescribed
three nourishing meals per day and a between-meal milkshake

designed to build lean muscle and supply him with energy. The shake contained vanilla Ensure, pure carbohydrate powder, Personal Edge soy protein powder, and Phosphocreatine, which I sometimes use to help athletes gain muscle mass with medical approval.

Within a few months the mayor went through a metamorphosis, experiencing a dramatic reduction in his symptoms. He gained fifteen pounds of lean muscle, became stronger, and regained his balance and energy. He has not only been able to do superlative work, but has also gone out and tackled some of the larger issues facing the city. In the ensuing months, he continued to see improvements in his health and well-being, resulting in more lean muscle, and energy. He recommended my wellness program to his four hundred city employees, and so far, over a hundred of them have signed up.

Just as I help athletes in the arena of competitive sports to extend their careers far beyond what they formerly believed was possible, I also teach my business athletes, the ordinary men and women with whom I work, how to achieve exceptional levels of health and fitness for life. In this book you will find everything you need to know to reduce your health age far below your chronological age. With proper lifestyle management, any man or woman can remain in their prime at the peak of their experience and achieve high performance in all areas of life.

Secret 2: Reduce Your Fatigue Threshold

Managing fatigue and reducing your fatigue threshold are essential to maintaining maximum performance. No one can work at peak efficiency when he or she is exhausted all the time. According to Dr. Hans Seyle, a leading stress researcher, we all have an energetic savings account and a checking account. If you consistently overdraw your energetic checking account—your daily energy reserves—through overwork, unmanaged stress, and ignored health warnings, eventually your checking account will empty and you will have to draw on your savings account—the body's emergency energy reserves.

Twelve years ago Lomas Brown, an NFL player on the offensive line for the Detroit Lions, came to me because he was having problems with his knee joints. Since the NFL is always looking for bigger, stronger, and faster linemen, Lomas's weight was 310 pounds. When

I ran him through our health checks, I discovered that his Body Mass Index and his body fat composition were much too high.

At this point, Lomas had already played eight years on the defensive line. He knew that he didn't have the energy of a rookie anymore. He wanted to improve his performance so he could stay in the game for a few more years, but he couldn't do this unless something changed for him. He also knew that overweight offensive and defensive linemen had a 50 percent greater chance of dropping dead of a heart attack than the average man on the street. He wanted to be around to enjoy his children and his grandchildren when his career was over.

Since Lomas was a seasoned veteran with some of the best technique I'd ever seen, there was only one suggestion I could make. I told him, "Since the quickest way to compromise technique is to become tired out, let's work on improving your fatigue threshold by dropping your weight and getting you better conditioned."

Soon we had his weight down to 280 pounds, with more lean muscle and less body fat. But then Lomas said, "Mackie, that's all fine and good, but my offensive lineman coach wants me to weigh in at 295."

I said, "But you've also had knee surgery. Increasing your weight will be harder on your knees in the long run, so I think we'll have to keep your weight down lower if you want to achieve your goal. Talk to your agent. Tell him 'When I go into the preseason training camp, weigh me in at 295 automatically. Let my statistics speak for me. If I do what I need to do, then my coach can just assume I'm 295 pounds.'"

Lomas followed this advice and became all-pro that year. He's been all-pro for a total of nine seasons. At a final weight of 276 pounds, he became the lightest player in the NFL at left tackle. When he first came to me, he only wanted to squeeze another three years out of his career. But he got an additional nine, as one of the highest paid left tackles in the game—and he's still playing as of this writing. He learned how to improve his performance by managing his fatigue.

Since you are born with only a limited amount of energy, the key to maintaining a high level of performance and productivity is learning how to *manage* that energy. There are several ways to do this:

- Your heart has only a finite number of beats in it before it stops forever, but you do not have to squander those beats because your aerobic conditioning is poor. Through exercise, you can always develop a lower resting heart rate.

- Get regular health checkups.
- Make sure you get enough sleep.
- Keep your weight within acceptable limits.
- Manage your stress (see chapter 6).

Secret 3: Manage Your Performance to Go the Distance

One of the keys to delivering maximum performance is being able to manage your energy so that you can go the distance. Every task takes a certain amount of time, and you must maintain enough energy during that time to effectively exercise your skills, talents, judgment, and teamwork long enough so that you can win. Athletes are great role models for energy management. For example, boxers must be able to control their energy expenditures for twelve rounds. It does not matter if you give your opponent the battle of his life for five rounds if you don't have the stamina to finish the fight. The workplace is no different. To complete a task or a project, you need to be able to go the distance.

The competitive challenge in life as in sports is to maintain your own energy levels while pushing your opponent into a state of overuse and overreaching. On the other hand, wise energy management involves being smart enough to never allow others to maneuver you into a position where *you* are being forced to overreach, to attempt a task that you know is beyond what you can realistically do. That could automatically set you up for a failure.

- *Always perform with integrity.* If you have integrity, you will go the distance with your client, even when the chips are down. You will stand by your people, handle and minimize the damage, cut your losses, analyze what went wrong, and create a better plan to help you make a comeback.
- *Never overreach yourself.* Managing your energy system is crucial to going the distance. It does not matter how much sheer talent and experience you have if you are overreaching. Whatever amount of energy you are putting out daily on your job,

make sure that it is never so much that you are not able to recover.

The upside of the equation is that once you have learned how to manage your energy system, you are almost always going to be able to go the distance and accomplish whatever performance goals you set for yourself.

Secret 4: Control Your Emotions for Maximum Performance

Being in control of your emotions at all times is another important key to maximum performance. Controlling your emotions is not the same thing as suppressing them. Rather, I'm referring to a technique that will allow your emotions to easily pass through you as they happen so that you will not become so emotionally paralyzed, stressed, or unfocused that you cannot perform properly. If you cannot gain access to your emotions, acknowledge them, and process them, you lose energy because they move below the conscious level and become tied up somewhere inside, creating an energetic short circuit. The result is compromised performance.

In order to keep that short circuit from happening every time you encounter an emotional stressor, utilize an autohypnosis technique: Squeeze your hand into a fist and release it five times, repeating the word *control* and consciously letting go of the stressor. Each time you do this, simply feel your emotions and your stress pass through you. Sometimes it helps to visualize your heart in your hand and to see yourself squeezing out the tension and gently releasing it.

Emotional equilibrium is key to achieving high performance.

Secret 5: Keep Your Work Life and Your Personal Life Balanced

Many people lose sight of the fact that it is just as important to perform well at home as it is at work. What good is performing hard at work for those you love if you never have any time to spend with them? And how long would you expect a family member, friend, or significant other to stay in your life if you are never around? Personal relationships might be the reason you work long hours, but you must ask yourself, Have I been mindful enough to arrange my work load and my personal life in such a way that they are in balance? Or has my life become lopsided?

My wife Sandy works daily to keep a healthy balance between the demands of her career and of being a wife and mother of two. Sandy is the president and CEO of the New Orleans Tourism Marketing Corporation. Since tourism is the number one industry in New Orleans and involves 65,000 jobs, this position is tremendously demanding. She must coordinate the activities of her corporation with two others—the Convention and Visitors' Bureau and the New Orleans Hotel/Motel Association—as well as answer to both a high-powered board of directors and to the city counsel of New Orleans while she manages a budget of roughly $10 million.

Following the terrorist attacks of September 11, 2001—when tourism had almost stopped due to fear of flying—Sandy came up with a campaign called "New Orleans on a Song." Anyone who drove to the city and stayed two nights would receive a third night at their hotel free. It took quite a bit of hard work, cooperation, and quick planning, but the campaign was successful and tourism began to pick up again. In a city that depends so much on tourism, this was welcome news.

But no matter how hard the job gets, Sandy always manages to spend a good deal of time with her family. The secrets of her success are organization, always looking ahead to see what is going to be happening with the family, and working closely with me and others to meet the needs of our children and ensure that our home runs smoothly. On Sunday nights, Sandy creates a calendar for the week describing all the kids' school and sports activities, when they will occur and where. One copy goes to me and one goes on the kitchen bulletin board. In this way, everyone knows what is coming up and how to plan ahead.

Sandy and I have always known how important it is for the two of us to work together to keep our home life balanced and our kids'—and our own—needs met. We share grocery shopping and cooking the meals. Both of us try, whenever possible, to be present at important functions at the school, but if one of us is not available, we make sure that the other is.

If you can focus, communicate, and plan ahead, you can achieve balance between maximum performance in a successful career and loving performance in your home life.

Secret 6: Learn to Anticipate Life's Next Moves

Another aspect of maximum performance is being able to anticipate your opponent's next moves. If you do then you need only take the actions most needed, and you will not waste precious energy rushing around trying this, that, and the other thing until you get it right. Great athletes know how to enhance their performance through anticipating the competition. Retired Miami Dolphin Dan Marino could always come up to the line of scrimmage and have a very accurate idea of where his opponents were going to move. Wayne Gretsky, one of the greatest hockey players of all time, could always see the puck coming two moves away. He knew so much about his game and the people he played against that he could almost always guess what the opposition—and his fellow teammates—were going to do next. Tiger Woods has the same gift.

In life, we need not only to be aware of what's going on in the here and now but also to be able to look down the road and see what's approaching. Some blows are inevitable, and the best we can do is to see them coming and try to limit the damage. Others we can prepare for so that we don't *have to* sustain damage.

General George S. Patton once wrote: "I have studied the enemy all my life. I have read the memoirs of his generals and his leaders. I have even read his philosophers and listened to his music. I have studied in great detail the account of every damned one of his battles. I know exactly how he will react under any given set of circumstances."

All of us need to learn how to patiently study and understand those we compete against in life and in the workplace. Always focus on the big picture and anticipate the future. Some tips for doing this include:

- Head off the younger, less experienced coworker who is after your job.
- Read the signs of your industry and see when things are going to make a downturn or a major shift—and be ready.
- See that tremendous opportunity down the road and position yourself so that you are ready to grasp it when it presents itself to you.
- Never become complacent in your career or in any other area of your life. Educate yourself about new developments in your field and make yourself available for new training opportunities.

- Seek out willing mentors who can honestly evaluate your skills and teach you things you could never learn otherwise.

The ability to look ahead and accurately foresee the next move will give you a performance edge that those who spend their lives rushing around to catch up just won't be able to match.

Secret 7: Perform Well to Your Last Breath

There is no overtime in life. Therefore it benefits us to perform with as much gusto as we can until our very last breath.

In a very real sense, the adversary all of us will eventually face is death. For this reason a question you must ask yourself is, How do I want to die? Do you want to end up living in a nursing home for the last decade of your life because you can no longer take care of yourself? Do you want to spend your final years partially paralyzed by a stroke? Would you look forward to the pain and limited mobility of arthritis or the hassle of having to replace a knee or hip because the joint was just worn out by overuse or abuse? Would you enjoy being extremely overweight and suffering from obesity-related illnesses such as type 2 diabetes and heart disease?

Or do you want to enjoy life, playing and working for as many years as possible?

I often ask my clients, "If how you live is determined by how you want to die, what performance strategies must you develop to work and live with gusto?" While the average life span for men is seventy-eight and for women is eighty-two, that figure has been steadily increasing. In fact researchers are projecting that by the year 2025, sixty-two million people will be over the age of sixty-five, and by 2040 as many as one million people will celebrate their hundredth birthday. Many of us will live much longer than our parents did.

The choice we face is this: Do we want to spend our later years as a drain on society, suffering from health problems that are largely avoidable? Or do we want to remain a good prospect for as long as possible, performing with energy and a zest for life?

Dr. Christiaan Barnard, the physician who did the first heart transplant, said, "I want to die 'young' as late as possible." I love to share this with my clients. When I repeated this to one woman, she told me, "That reminds me of my Great Aunt Ruth. She always walked everywhere—miles and miles per week, ate right, and kept her joy for living alive by traveling the world with her children and cultivating friends of all ages. She ran her own business, retired, then managed to keep active and live independently all the way up to the age of ninety-one. At that point she had a stroke that partially paralyzed her and put her into a nursing home. The last eight months of her life were hard for all of us, but at least we knew that she had lived the first ninety-one years with good health and gusto."

There is no overtime in life, no going back onto the field for one last play. The lifestyle choices we make every day truly determine the level of our performance, whether we remain a good prospect or become suspect. It's up to us to make sure we're choosing wisely.

3

Nine Strategies to
Achieve Your Goals

Setting goals is the only way to insure that you will keep moving toward the things you wish to achieve in life. Unfortunately, many people set goals only to be bitterly disappointed when they fail to reach them, time and time again. What are the secrets to reaching your goals and attaining your dreams?

Before you begin, I suggest you take this brief questionnaire. It will help you to evaluate your present goal-setting style. Check "never," "sometimes," or "always."

Questionnaire: How Do You Approach Goal Setting?

	Never	Some-times	Always
1. I let the opinions of others influence what goals I set and my confidence about whether I can reach them.	☐	☐	☐
2. Before setting a new goal, I thoroughly evaluate where I am at this moment.	☐	☐	☐
3. When I set goals, I know where I want to go in the long run.	☐	☐	☐
4. I have a clear picture of where I want to end up when I set my goals.	☐	☐	☐
5. I plan out my goals in incremental steps.	☐	☐	☐
6. I feel relaxed and clearheaded when thinking about my goals.	☐	☐	☐

During my twenty-five years of work with thousands of professional athletes and ordinary people from all walks of life, I have discovered that there are nine basic concepts behind achieving your goals. These strategies will enable you to discover where you are now, what you really want to achieve, how to get yourself there, and how to stay there once you have achieved your current goal.

Strategy 1: Don't Allow Others to Say You Cannot Achieve Your Goal

Brett Butler's recovery from cancer and miraculous return to baseball is a prime example of this. Few of us have goals as dramatic and as crucial as his—to beat the disease that had undermined his strength and his health and to play the game he loved again, in spite of the fact that his doctors believed he probably never would. His journey is one of the most inspiring in which I have ever had the privilege to participate and is an example of what we can achieve when we refuse to give up.

In May 1996, Brett had fifty lymph nodes removed from his neck and throat. One of them was cancerous. Since I had worked with him for the last eight years and was a close friend, I was one of the first people that Brett called when he learned about his cancer. He was well aware of the many athletes with serious injuries and health problems whom I had helped make a comeback, such as Tulane University baseball player Jared Robinson, who tore up his shoulder so badly that the doctors said he'd never throw again. Jared focused on his recovery with unwavering determination and did everything I told him to do. In no time at all, he was back, pitching better than ever.

Brett's ultimate goal was to live, but to him that meant being able to play baseball again. He told me that he had to get back because being out on that baseball diamond was life itself to him. I told him I'd do everything in my power to help him.

The first thing we did was assess exactly Brett's health and what his doctors were saying about his prospects for making a full recovery. This is tough to do with cancer because it's impossible to get a scouting report on it, as you can for a human opponent. But we also knew three things right from the start: (1) Brett was a man who had tremendous faith and a solid belief system; (2) he was a fighter; and (3) we had two great allies—traditional medicine and alternative medicine—and we knew we could make them work well together, complementing each other.

We began by breaking down Brett's goal into small steps, creating a strategic plan that would enable us to learn everything we could about his cancer, both past and present. The first decision we had to make was whether Brett would have chemotherapy as well as radiation treatment. He opted not to have the chemo, since it would increase his life expectancy by only 5 percent and would seriously depress his immune system, which had been a weakness with him for many years. Brett had perennially suffered from tonsil-related viruses and Epstein-Barr, a type of chronic fatigue syndrome. Since he had taken antibiotics for prolonged periods of time, much of the "good" bacteria in his large intestine had regularly been killed off. Since much of immune function is based on a healthy large intestine, we didn't want to weaken him further.

When we showed Brett's medical report to Dr. James Carter, emeritus chairperson of the Nutrition Section at the Tulane University School of Public Health and Tropical Medicine and an alternative- and preventative-medicine specialist, he said, "I don't think this is simply cancer of the tonsils. There is something much deeper at work. Let's send a sample of his biopsy to a special lab." When the lab report came back, there were traces of the Epstein-Barr virus in the tumor itself, leading Dr. Carter to conclude that there was a direct link between the cancer and Brett's weakened immune system.

One of our first goals, then, was to do everything in our power to strengthen Brett's immune system. I called on Dr. Charlie Brown, a team physician for the New Orleans Saints and a cancer specialist, to chart Brett's white blood cell count, monitor his progress, and do everything for him that traditional medicine could possibly do. Brett took the usual course of radiation treatments recommended for someone in his condition (thirty-two in all), but at the same time he also decided to receive care and medications from American Biologics, a medical clinic in Tijuana, Mexico, that specializes in alternative treatments for cancer patients. Dr. Carter agreed to administer and monitor the protocols prescribed by doctors at that clinic, which included IV drips of amino acids, vitamin C, and other nutrients.

Another important step toward Brett's recovery was to build his weight back up. At five foot nine, he normally weighed 165 pounds. During his illness he had lost 20 pounds of muscle. He looked emaciated and felt weak. I had plenty of experience helping people to gain needed weight, since I had worked with many tall thin NBA players who burned off the pounds during the basketball season. With Brett, however, there was an additional problem. After his radiation treatments his throat was swollen and covered with sores. How were we going to build him back up if he couldn't swallow enough solid food?

We found part of our answer one afternoon when we were sitting in the doctors' dining room at the hospital. A radiologist at our table said, "When we have to desensitize the throat to put something down it, such as a tube, we numb the throat with a special medication." I asked him if he would call the pharmacist and order some of this for Brett. He agreed, and Brett began gargling with the medication before meals. It worked perfectly, and he was able to swallow food again without pain.

We also created a special drink for Brett to aid in his weight gain. This consisted of vanilla Ensure, a high-carbohydrate powder called Carboplex, creatine monohydrate to increase his muscle mass, and Personal Edge soy protein powder. Brett drank this three times a day between meals and slowly began to gain back the weight he had lost.

Once Brett became strong enough to begin exercising again, I created a special resistance-training program for him. Since his surgery had left him with impaired nerve function, I hooked up his shoulder to a monitor to make sure that we were not overtiring his nerves or his muscles. I also got him back into baseball-related activities. The New Orleans Zephyrs gave him permission to do batting practice with them.

Meanwhile his family came and stayed at the Windsor Court Hotel in New Orleans so that he could go "home" to them at the end of the day instead of having to be far away from the people who were most important to him during his recovery.

The results of all these factors were remarkable. Brett gained back seventeen pounds of muscle in twenty-three days, and over a six-week period, his immune function and all of his blood levels improved dramatically. He was able to return to his team, open the series in Montreal, then return back home to a standing ovation in Dodgers' Stadium. He scored the winning run that night. Sports commentators referred to that season as "the amazing comeback." Brett eventually wrote about his recovery in a book called *Field of Hope,* in which he devoted an entire chapter to the work we had done together. As of this writing he is still cancer free.

Strategy 2: Evaluate Where You Are at This Point

Before you set any goal it is a good idea to evaluate yourself, your talents, and your desires as thoroughly as possible. This will help you not only to achieve your goal, but also to avoid wasting energy pursuing a goal you are not really suited for. Sometimes people choose goals that are not a good match for their abilities. For example, I've met several men and women who decided to put themselves through the arduous training of law school because that profession has prestige and great financial rewards. But although they earned their degrees with honors, when they actually began to practice, they discovered that they didn't like being a lawyer. Lawyers have to fight, to be aggressive, to look at negatives, and to pick everything apart. If you don't have a forceful personality that feels challenged by conflict and loves a good legal battle, it's difficult to last long in that profession.

If you believe you want to do something but are unsure whether that is the correct goal for you, seek out the opinion of people you trust. Get feedback from coworkers, friends, and mentors that you respect. Others can often see your strengths and weaknesses more clearly than you can see them yourself. Sitting down with a piece of paper and making a list of pros and cons is always helpful in selecting and refining your goal.

Strategy 3: Know Where You Want to Go in the Long Run

Brett Butler's goal was not only to survive cancer by getting the best treatment possible, but he also wanted to get back to the game of baseball because that was where he felt most alive. Every choice he made, every step of the way, was focused on getting back onto the field of his dreams.

The more clearly you can visualize your long-term goals, the more likely you are to avoid wasting your time and energy reaching them. For example, if your goal is to spend your life working as a healer who eases people's suffering, training to be a medical doctor might be the best way to achieve that goal—or it might leave you feeling frustrated and disillusioned. The pressures on doctors are intense in the "write-and-rip" world of the modern HMO, where they will see dozens of patients a day. Some doctors who work in that system find ways to remain emotionally connected and caring toward their patients. Others become so stressed by its demands that they become emotionally disconnected or addicted to prescription drugs to keep themselves going. There are a hundred ways to become a healer, both traditional and nontraditional. The trick is figuring out what kind of person *you* are and in what sort of world you would feel most comfortable and fulfilled.

There are many ways of achieving your goals once you know where you want to be in the long run. Looking down the road and clearly visualizing the work, relationship, or promotion that you really want can save you from being disappointed and wasting your energy.

Strategy 4: Use Dreams and Visualizations to See Yourself There

As you work toward your goal, always spend a certain amount of time each day actually *seeing* your goal as an accomplished fact. Visualize what it would feel like to be there, doing what you dream about doing. Picture yourself with that promotion, that book deal, that award, that degree. If you are training for the marathon, see yourself running, passing other runners, crossing the finish line with the best time you've ever achieved. If your goal is to lose weight or put on more muscle, visualize that during your workout. Feel yourself becoming stronger, the waistline of your pants becoming looser. Hear those compliments from your friends and family about how good you look. See your heart become stronger.

Daily meditation will also help you to visualize your goal. Once you are completely relaxed, imagine yourself in your goal and watch what happens. Often, the scene will play itself out like a movie and you will learn valuable information about your goal. You may want to keep a notebook handy to write down what you see.

Strategy 5: Make Incremental Steps Toward Your Goal

The place where a lot of people go wrong is not knowing how to break their goals down into logical, attainable steps. Any long-term goal must be reached in smaller stages. Begin by evaluating where you are in the present in relationship to where you want to be in the future. Then, based on your skills, talents, emotional stability, and level of preparation, begin exploring what, for you, would be a realistic and desirable goal. Once you know where you want to go in the long run, you can begin to plan step 1, step 2, and so forth. By taking small steps you often can go further down the road than you ever hoped to go, achieving things that you originally felt were beyond you.

A forty-seven-year-old friend of mine named Angela realized that she had been steadily putting on weight since she turned forty. Angela had always been physically active when she was in her twenties and thirties. She had jogged regularly, taken yoga and dance classes, and enjoyed ballroom dancing. As with so many of us, however, her activity level began to drop off as she got older. In the last decade, she had begun writing professionally, work that forced her to be sedentary for most of the day.

When Angela was given the opportunity to ghostwrite a book with a nutritionist and fitness professional, she saw this as a chance to take off her unwanted weight and get into better physical condition. At five feet eight inches, she weighed 158 pounds. She had never been overweight before, and she wanted to reverse this trend before it became a problem. Her goal was to lose twenty pounds.

When the nutritionist gave her a complimentary health evaluation to get a clear picture of her present overall health, Angela was surprised by the results. Normally, a total cholesterol level of 200 is considered borderline healthy. Angela's was 193, although this was balanced somewhat by her HDL (good cholesterol) of 72, almost twice the acceptable amount. Her triglycerides were good at 98. This was all in keeping with the new guidelines developed by the American College of Cardiology that state that a woman's total cholesterol should never be higher than 200 mg/dl, her HDL should never fall below 50 mg/dl, and her triglycerides should never exceed 150.

But the shocker was her body fat percentage, a whopping 34.5 percent! Suddenly she realized that she was not just twenty pounds overweight, she was technically obese, since a healthy woman her age should have a body fat percentage between 18 and 23 percent. She not only had to lose weight, but she also had to build back more lean muscle.

Like many people trying to lose weight, Angela discovered that she was eating less food than was optimal for her, about two-thirds of the total number of calories her body needed to maintain her metabolism. That meant that she had to actually begin eating *more food* in order to make her body efficient enough to lose fat and gain lean muscle. Perceiving that a famine was on, her body had been hoarding fat to protect itself.

Angela began following a food program the nutritionist designed for her, tailored to her individual needs. She began eating three balanced meals per day and two snacks to keep her metabolism working efficiently. She also made time in her schedule to begin exercising again. She began by walking between forty-five minutes to an hour every day. Within a month, her total cholesterol had dropped to 174 and her triglycerides to 60.

At this time I gave Angela a copy of my book *Lose Your Love Handles: A 3-Step Program to Streamline Your Waist in 30 Days*. Even though this book was written for men, Angela was tremendously impressed with it and began to add exercises for the core area of the body to her program. She was deeply gratified when her waistline became smaller and her abdominal muscles tighter. Most important, as she strengthened the muscles that held her spine in place, her back stopped hurting for the first time in years. She told me that she had resigned herself to having backaches as a part of the process of getting older. She was happy when I assured her this wasn't true.

After three months, Angela's weight had dropped to 140 pounds and her body fat to 25 percent. Since fat is three times the size of lean muscle, she looked much slimmer and more compact. In every sense, she had successfully achieved her goal of losing weight, gaining lean muscle, and becoming healthier. Her cholesterol was an amazing 137, with an HDL of 68; her triglycerides were a superefficient 52; and she had tons of energy. All her friends remarked about how good she looked.

At this point, Angela asked herself, If I can achieve this goal, why can't I do more? She had been somewhat sporadic about going to the gym, even though she had been faithful to her cardiovascular program of walking. Now she set a further goal of seeing if she could get her weight down to 135 pounds and decrease her body fat percentage even more. To accomplish this, she added faithful workouts in the gym three times a week to her program and asked me questions about supplements and improving her exercise program, which I gladly answered. As of this writing, Angela weighs 136 pounds and has dropped her body fat percentage to 20 percent. Her new goal is to weigh 125 pounds and have a body fat percentage of 16 percent. With the knowledge she has gained about exercise, nutrition, and weight loss, I have no doubt at all that she will get there.

Angela has realized something that I often tell my clients: your health age does not have to be the same as your chronological age. She is currently healthier, stronger, and more youthful than most women in their late forties, and she is eager to see where she can go next. Most important, she was able to achieve her goal because she took small realistic steps. If her goal had been to lose ten pounds in a week, she would have failed. Her clear vision of where she wanted to be at each stage, her careful research and planning about how to achieve each stage, and her incremental successes along the way sustained her motivation and kept her goal for greater health and fitness burning bright.

Strategy 6: Anticipate the Competition and Your Opponent's Strategy

In the world of sports, this is called getting a scouting report, finding out all you can about the team or other player you will be competing against. For example, in the NFL every Monday the team members watch films of the team they're going to play. These films are broken down into "positions" so that each man gets to watch the specific players he will be up against, learning their tendencies, studying every move they make.

Whatever your goal, it is necessary to learn everything you can about your opponent. Research his habits and strategies. Ask yourself how you can use your own strengths and abilities to remove any obstacles he may put in front of you. Be able to see two moves ahead. If you truly understand your opponent, you will be able to use that knowledge against him, leading him down the garden path of his expectations while actually lining him up so that you can knock him down with an unexpected move.

Strategy 7: Develop a Strategy for Distracting the Competition Long Enough to Give You an Opening or Advantage

One of the greatest strengths any person has is his or her instinct. A person who works from experience and instinct will invariably make the appropriate move. So if you can distract your opponents, forcing them to stop moving forward and start second-guessing themselves right in the middle of a negotiation or an important meeting, you will have put them at a distinct disadvantage.

A heavyweight champion I trained made this work for him in the boxing ring. His objective was to learn everything he could about his opponents' strategies so that he could lull them into feeling comfortable in the ring. He knew that once they became comfortable enough to think they were winning, they would lose their edge and begin to let down their guard. When he saw his opening, he would suddenly switch strategies and take them down.

We used this tactic when my client was getting ready to defend his heavyweight title against an opponent. His opponent was a big man who liked to intimidate people with his size—he was six feet five inches and 260 pounds to my client's six feet three inches and 205 pounds. The opponent also liked to talk about his strength and to be photographed lifting 300-pound barbells and doing neck exercises with excessively heavy weights, bragging that he was too tough to be knocked out.

My client was more worried about this fight than he had been about his first heavyweight fight. Since my client was really a "manufactured heavyweight," someone who'd moved up from the light heavyweight division, he was worried that he was about to lose it all to a guy who outweighed him by fifty-five pounds. We had to find a way to distract his opponent and give my client the opening he needed to defeat him.

I began by telling my fighter the story of the Trojan horse, how the Greeks had lulled the Trojans into thinking they were winning by seeming to stand down from the fight and wheel in a peace offering. In this way they deceived the Trojans into lowering their defenses. I told him that the secret to winning this fight was to wheel in his own Trojan horse by manipulating his opponent's perception both before and during the fight. We began by playing to his opponent's ego, having my client act as if he were awed by his opponent's great size. In all of his prefight interviews, my client made sure he talked about how strong and powerful his opponent was. We wanted to plant the idea in the other fighter's mind that he could tire out my client by coming on strong in his attack.

At the same time I worked on my client's stamina, giving him a competitive advantage by preparing him to deliver a barrage of fast and hard punches whenever he had his opening and then to move out of the way quickly to avoid getting hit when his opponent came back at him. By giving him greater stamina, we also gave him an enhanced ability to recover during the fight.

By the day of the fight, we had already wheeled our Trojan horse, my client's hypothetical awe of his opponent's size, into the ring. We hoped we had succeeded in making his opponent feel comfortable enough and sure enough of his victory that he would not ration his strength to last ten rounds, but would squander it, believing he could win early on in the fight. Sure enough, the opposition came on hard, wasting his strength and his punches, but I had trained my client to avoid most of them. Then in the sixth round the other fighter tried to get my client against the ropes, believing he now had him cornered and could finish him off, since he thought my client was intimidated by his great strength.

At that moment my boxer saw his opening and made his move by playing off the ropes. When his opponent came in to finish the fight, my client pivoted on him and hit him with a crashing blow to the right side of the head. If the referee hadn't stopped the fight, my client might have seriously injured the other fighter because I had conditioned him to keep going and fight until the end once he saw his opening.

When you can lull your opponent into his comfort zone by understanding his character and motivation and by manipulating his impression of you and your intentions, you can make the unexpected move when he lets down his offenses.

Strategy 8: Develop the Instinct to Make the Lateral Move When the Punch Is Coming So That You Don't Get Hurt

No one can ever control all of the variables of life and business. There are times when life delivers an unexpected disappointment, no matter how much you have studied and planned. At such times you must act with dignity and be coolheaded, learning your lessons, letting go of defeat, and turning your energy and attention toward new goals and possibilities. You must also learn how to cut your losses and minimize the damage so you can protect yourself and your colleagues.

One of the most effective ways I have found to make a lateral move is to go against type, to act in a different manner than your opponent expects you to. This behavior will also stop your opponents in their tracks, making them wonder, "What in the world is he/she doing? I thought I knew what was going to happen today. Now I'm not so sure." Building an unexpected move into your strategy throws an opponent off balance, buying you valuable time to make your move.

People relate to you based on what they believe about you—their perception of you—and they always expect you to act predictably, because that is human nature. "She's a thinker, so she's going to take the intellectual approach to this problem." "He's outgoing, energetic, and easily excitable. I can throw him off balance if I get him worked up." "She's more of a risk taker than any man in the office—jumps in where others fear to tread. If I can get her to go too far out on a limb, I've got her." "He moves slowly and carefully—never makes a decision until he's analyzed the situation from every angle. I can throw him off balance if I force him to move more quickly than he feels comfortable doing."

Making a lateral move involves developing strategies and ways of operating that run contrary to the way the world perceives you. You will also develop ways to think on your feet when someone throws you a curve and intuitively choose an effective course of action.

Strategy 9: Learn to Relax

One of the most important things you can do in life and in business is to learn how to relax, especially in situations when the proverbial heat is on. You need peace of mind to be creative and productive. When you try to create under duress, that's really reaction, not creation. The first thing I did when I had a crisis situation in a meeting with an oil company, to which I had proposed a corporate health program, was to put my hand down under the table, squeeze my fist five times, and repeat to myself, Control, control, control. Next, I separated myself from the situation and focused on putting things into perspective. This meeting occurred shortly after the terrorist attacks on the World Trade Center and the Pentagon. Even though things at the meeting had not turned out the way I wanted them to, I realized that my disappointment was small compared to the problems that many other people were facing that week. I thought to myself, There are a lot of people out there who just lost their lives and there are policemen, fire fighters, and rescue workers out there trying to save people. In the scope of things, this one disappointment doesn't amount to a hill of beans. Then I let it all go. Instead of reacting in anger and frustration and giving those people a piece of my mind, I left the meeting thinking about how to create closure with as much integrity and dignity as I could. In the days to come, I did not sit around brooding and feeling angry. I focused my creative energy on the other projects I was developing.

Learning to relax in the face of stress, conflict, or defeat is all about perspective. When you know that the situation has changed and the battle is lost, don't waste energy fighting for a lost cause. If you can, shift the battle to your own territory, as I did with the oil company, forcing them to come onto my own turf and pay full price for the program if they still wanted it. But if you can't do that, cut your losses. Move on to the next project.

When you make your goals as clear as possible by breaking them down into manageable steps, and understand the competition so you know how to get out of the way when you see the hard punches coming, you will always come away from your public and personal battles with a sense of accomplishment and the knowledge that you have learned and achieved something valuable.

4

Discover and Balance
Your Energy Style

The first step toward learning how to manage your performance is to determine how you *personally* use energy, because we are not all alike. We all have a different energy utilization styles. I have found that most people fall within one of two categories: the type A and the type B personality.

We've all met people who are boisterous, outgoing, and overdramatic. This is the type A personality. The positive aspect of this personality is that those who have it are energizing and inspiring to be around. The downside is that they can use more energy than needed to complete a task and burn themselves out.

The type B personality includes people who live very much in their heads. They are introspective. At their best, they are great planners and organizers. At their worst, they fritter away their energy by worrying about everything. Often they need external motivation.

As your read the descriptions below, keep in mind that while each of us has a strong *tendency* to be either one type or the other, depending on how we habitually deal with life, no one is type A or type B 100 percent of the time. These two types are meant as guidelines to help you evaluate what you are in the *present moment* so that you can learn how to modify your energy utilization curve. Whether you are experiencing the intense energy of the type A or the slower, more introspective pace of the type B, keep in mind

39

that your ultimate goal should always be to *balance* your energy to help you deal more effectively with any situation in which you find yourself.

The Type A Personality

A typical type A personality works from his sympathetic nervous system (fight or flight) and wastes energy by always being in overdrive. His motto is "Okay, let's go!" and he will often find something to keep him busy even when the task at hand is finished. He can be his own worst enemy because he is always wearing himself out. When he talks, he breathes shallowly and uses short, choppy sentences. I think of type A personalities as "interval" people because they do everything quick and fast. They jump rapidly from task to task and from thought to thought.

High-energy professions tend to attract type A personalities. I know an ophthalmologist who is type A. She is in a constant state of activity, seeing fifty patients a day, moving from room to room, and writing up reports. When this individual speaks with me, her voice is breathy and her words staccato because her breathing pattern is quick and shallow, coming from the top third of her lungs. Her sentences are short and choppy. A side effect of this quick, shallow breathing and these overblown emotions is an overproduction of acid in her stomach. Every day of her life she takes Prilosec tablets for her acid reflux.

The Type B Personality

The type B personality, who works from the parasympathetic nervous system (the relaxation response), is always worrying about everything. This kind of person is always sighing and saying, "Oh, man, what am I going to do? How are we going to get this done on time?" You can literally hear the air escaping from his lungs. By the time he goes into the business meeting, he's totally worn himself out by imagining every possible scenario over and over in his head. He hardly has any energy left for the actual task at hand. If the type A personality does everything in intervals, the type B personality doesn't tend to jump from one thing to the next. He just feels overwhelmed and at loose ends.

Five Steps to Help Balance Your Type A Energy Style

If you are a type A personality, what can you do to bring yourself back into balance so that you are not constantly exploding with physical and emotional energy and burning yourself out? I suggest the following five steps:

1. *Slow your breathing.* Learn to listen to the sound of your own voice. When you hear the pitch going upward and feel your sentences getting more rushed or your words more staccato, deliberately slow down your speech. This will enable you to step back from a stressful situation, calm your thoughts, and achieve some emotional objectivity. While the person you are addressing is speaking, take a moment to inhale all the way down into your diaphragm on a slow count of two and exhale on a slow count of four. Connecting to a slow, steady, deep breath will slow down your heartbeat and give your nervous system a signal that it can pull back from the "fight or flight" syndrome. In other words, your body will know it is safe to relax.

2. *Speak in complete sentences.* Type A personalities often speak in incomplete sentences or jump from thought to thought. When this speaking pattern intensifies, consciously pull yourself back and make yourself take the time to speak in complete sentences. This will give your body the signal to slow down, breathe more deeply, and refocus.

3. *Increase dietary fiber.* Since this personality type usually produces more stomach acid, increase the fiber in your diet to give your stomach something to soak up that extra acid.

4. *Practice calming techniques.* Make time in your day to practice activities that dissipate stress, calm your nervous system, slow down your heartbeat, and help you to become more self-aware. This includes activities such as meditation, yoga, biofeedback, and visualization. If you can learn how to meditate and visualize effectively, you can take yourself to a more calm setting in your imagination where your mind will be freer to come up with creative strategies for accomplishing your daily tasks. As time goes on, it will take less and less effort to achieve a sense of being centered and balanced when you feel yourself going into overdrive.

5. *Build "steady-state" behaviors into your lifestyle.* Since the type A personality does everything from speaking to working to thinking in short intervals, it is important for you to counterbalance that habitual behavior by adopting more activities that are "steady state," that is, longer in duration. A good way to start is to make time to walk every day. Walking is great because it keeps the body moving while allowing the mind to function at a more focused, relaxed pace. If you obsess about the office or your next project while walking, you will defeat your own purpose. Let this be a time out where you can admire the scenery, smell the roses, and become reacquainted with yourself. In other words, let your walking be more like meditating than running a marathon.

If you practice these five points, I guarantee that they will help you to balance out the energy of your type A personality and increase the efficiency of your performance at work. It might seem contradictory to say that slowing yourself down several times during the day will increase your productivity, but experience has taught me that a lifestyle based on constant frenetic activity soon reaches a point of diminishing returns.

Helping a Stressed-Out Coach Learn How to Relax

Many football coaches are classic type A personalities. You can hear it in the way they bark at players during the game. "Let's go. Do this. Get over there." You seldom hear them using complete sentences. They are always speaking in choppy intervals, taking short and shallow breaths. This kind of never-ending stress is hard on the body, causing weight gain and often heart problems.

One particular coach became overweight and developed colitis. Since this man was always in interval mode, I reconditioned his nervous system to remember what relaxation felt like. To accomplish this, I had him spend twenty minutes walking at a steady-state pace before every game so that he could get used to keeping his breathing deep and even. During the off season I had him work with other steady-state activities such as meditation. He not only began to handle the game better, but he also lost weight and handled his life better.

Five Steps to Balance Your Type B Energy Style

At its worst, the type B personality can be dreamy, unfocused, depressed, and filled with worries. Here are four steps to help bring yourself back into balance if you are a type B personality:

1. *Put the interval back into your life.* In other words, get yourself into a routine where you do things at a specific time. Wake up at the same time every day, exercise at the same time every day. Get creative about structuring your life so that you are filling your day with interesting activities.
2. *Put your worries into perspective.* Worrying about something is almost always far worse than the reality. If you are worried about something, such as your financial future, get the facts. Sit down with your accountant and find out exactly where you stand and what you can do to improve your financial position. Talk out your worries with a trusted friend or mentor. If you are a type B then you tend to live too much in your head, so get outside of the closed circuit of your own mind and obtain some perspective.
3. *Face your fears through action.* Type B personalities tend to spend too much time planning how they are going to accomplish the next challenging task. Needless procrastination will only increase your stress levels. There comes a point where you have to realize that over-planning can lead to paralysis. Know when to say "Enough thought!" and face your fears squarely by taking firm action.
4. *Create the interval in your exercise program.* Where the body goes, the mind will soon follow. If you usually walk two to three miles per day, alternate that with periods of running every other day. If you exercise at the gym, put more variety into your activities. Do ten minutes on a treadmill, ten minutes on a stationary bike, and ten minutes of rowing or climbing.

By restructuring your life so that you spend more time moving forward in short energetic bursts, you can balance the energy of your type B personality. A sigh of depression is not necessarily a sign of exhaustion. It is often a signal that your energy is blocked. Release your bottled-up energy by reintroducing your body and mind to the joy of movement and vitality.

Putting the Interval Back into a Golfer's Game

Recently, I helped a type B client who was a tremendously talented golfer. He would always do well at driving the ball to the green, but his performance fell off when it came to putting. The reason for this was because he worked himself up into such a state of tension from anxiety that he wore himself out and lost his focus. It got to where he began to consistently fall apart on the last day of any competition. This makes sense when you remember that type B personalities do well with steady-state activities but tend to have difficulty maintaining control of short bursts of energy.

In order to help him remain focused and keep his energy levels high, I began training him to work with the concept of "interval." I did this by having him run for thirty seconds (tension), then walk for thirty seconds (relaxation), then run for thirty seconds, then walk. In this way I reconditioned him by actually retraining his nervous system to automatically let go whenever he became tense. It worked, and his game improved.

Whether you are a type A or a type B, balancing your energy style will help you go the distance as well.

5

Minimize Your Fear and Maximize Your Focus

One of the most important tasks you must learn is to manage your fear. Everyone is afraid at one time or another. If you told me you didn't feel fear, I'd say you were lying. We are afraid of failure, afraid of not measuring up, afraid that our creative wellspring of ideas will run dry, afraid that the next Young Turk will come along and take away our job.

Fear can wear you down and sap your energy. When faced with fear, you have two choices: you can let it stop you, or you can move beyond it.

Fear Is a Matter of Perception

Many people do not realize that fear is based not so much on objective fact as it is on the way that we *perceive* ourselves and our situations. I clearly saw how perception affects fear when I put a heart monitor on two hockey players during a two-hour-and-forty-minute preseason practice session. The figures show their heart rates during that session. The dotted middle line drawn across the graph represents the median heart rate. The spikes represent the highest and lowest heart rates during the on-ice sessions. The low points in the graph represent time spent sitting on the bench, and the lowest points represent time out in the locker room between periods. The first graph is a young rookie defenseman who was trying to make the team and the second is a veteran defenseman who had been in the league for eight years.

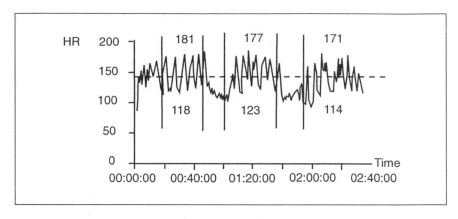

Rookie's heart rate. He has lots of energy but he gives it away; he's not sure how to get from point A to point B.

One of the first things you notice about the rookie defenseman is that his heart rate is more erratic than the veteran's. He starts at 100 beats per minute, goes up to 140 during the warm-up, then drops down to 118. During the first period his heart rate rises to 181, then drops to 118, and so on. The longer the practice, the more erratic his heart rate becomes and the more jagged his transitions.

When you look at the graph representing the veteran defenseman, you notice something different. No matter what quarter he's in, his heart rate glides up and down with tremendous consistency, showing how focused he is on the moment. Whereas the rookie has a 10-point difference in his highest heart rates in all three quarters, the veteran has only a 5-point difference. And each of the veteran's high points is so even, you could take a ruler and draw a straight line across the top of his chart. The same is true of the veteran's lowest heart rates. While the rookie's has a variance of 9 points, and is always higher than his original heartbeat of 100, the veteran's rate drops right back down to between 95 and 97 every time.

Clearly the difference between the players is one of heart rate variability due to perception. The rookie has to deal with fear about his performance. If he doesn't play well for his team, he's gone, replaced by the next talented prospect. So while he has a lot of energy, he gives it all away by feeling anxious and expending too much energy on each task—because he's afraid of the consequences of failure.

The veteran, however, has confidence in his skill and knowledge and has learned how to manage his fear, using only the energy neces-

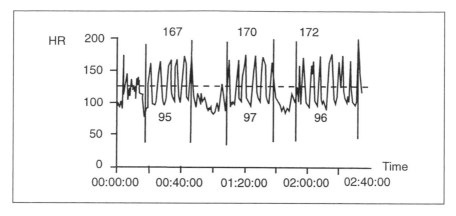

Heart rate of a veteran. He has less energy but much more stability; he takes things in their stride.

sary to deliver a good performance. He has innate knowledge and technique based on his experience curves, which permits him to accomplish each task in a much shorter period of time. The rookie's heart rate fluctuates erratically under pressure, giving away precious energy, but the veteran knows how to take the heat because he has learned with experience to manage his stress. At the end of the practice, the rookie is worn out. All he can think about is going home and going to bed. The veteran is getting ready to head out to the golf course.

The concept that fear is a matter of perception is even more clearly illustrated by the heart rate of the rookie goalie. Even though he's not involved in as much extended physical activity as his teammates, he feels the pressure not to let that hockey puck through. He is filled with anxiety, which drains him of energy. This player would lose twelve pounds per game because his nervousness made him sweat profusely. His heart would pound in anticipation of the next breakaway coming his way even when the other players were down at the far end of the ice.

If fear is a matter of perception, what tools can you use to learn how to manage it? How can you minimize your fear and maximize your focus?

You Can Change Your Perception

Fear is not a true indicator of danger but only of what we perceive to be happening. Often our perceptions are not based on reality. Many people have anxiety and panic attacks because they are imagining a scenario that never materializes. For example, some NFL players fear having to carry the ball too many times during the game because they know the statistics for getting injured go up dramatically the more you carry the ball.

The fear resulting from an inaccurate perception of a situation can turn you into your own worst enemy. Faced with a stressful situation, you will almost always imagine it to be much worse than it really is. Sitting on the sidelines and waiting to go into the game, the boardroom, or the meeting is much tougher than actually being in there performing. Too often you load yourself up with unnecessary apprehension, which threatens to weaken your performance. What can you do to manage fear and to help you be at the top of your form?

Prepare for a Specific Task

One way to conquer fear is to know that you have prepared yourself specifically for your task. This is done through conditioning and doing repetitions, not just with your body, but also with your mind. Then when you are finally called upon to perform, your experience and training will be able to take over, neutralizing your nervousness.

When I trained Michael Spinks, who was then a light heavyweight, to fight heavyweight champion Larry Holmes, I decided not to use the traditional methods of training boxers. Instead I focused on training Spinks for the actual tasks he would have to accomplish in the ring. Orthodox boxing training says that a fighter must go out and run five miles. But I knew that a boxing match is comprised of three minutes of fighting and one minute of rest. So I simulated those tasks by doing interval training. Michael and I ran for three minutes, then we rested for one minute.

It was so simple, but no one had thought to do it before. And it worked. After he won the championship against Larry, he told me our training methods truly simulated the fight conditions.

If you prepare specifically for your task, you will be able to manage your fear and be at your highest level of performance. There are many ways you might do this. For example:

- If you work in an office, keep abreast of new technologies in your field that will enable you to stay on top of your job.

- Volunteer for or request a special training program offered by your corporation, even if that means paying for this training session out of your own pocket.
- If you have a job that is highly people-oriented, or if you have received a promotion that places you in a position of leadership, review and refine your people management skills so that you can communicate with your team more clearly.

Sharpen Your Skills

A client of mine named Deborah is a systems analyst and programmer in the computer industry. Deborah is often asked to work on teams that include one or more people from out of town. These individuals are supposed to serve as conduits between her development team and the people at the site to which the software is headed.

During one such project, Deborah ended up with a woman on her team who seemed to feel that her status as a "visitor" meant that she didn't need to take the time or effort to be likeable or cooperative. Instead, her modus operandi was to issue curt orders to all of the software developers, to lose her temper when things weren't proceeding as she expected, and to generally act out in an abrasive and unpredictable manner. This behavior caused everyone on the team to feel unnecessary stress, fear, and loss of self-esteem. Because of these factors, the efficient functioning of the group and the smooth completion of the software development were jeopardized.

While looking for ways to improve this situation, Deborah discovered that her company offered its employees the Dale Carnegie course in developing self-confidence, communication, and confrontational skills. Since she was stuck with this uncooperative team member for the seven months of the project, she quickly availed herself of this program.

This training prepared Deborah for the specific task of completing her work on this project and restoring a measure of harmony to her team. One of the most important things Deborah learned was that we *allow* other people to walk all over us and destroy our confidence. This program enabled her:

- To regain her objectivity about herself and the situation.
- To learn valuable tools to help her work and communicate with people who manipulate others through anger and intimidation.

By regaining her self-confidence, Deborah learned how to manage her fear of her abrasive coworker effectively. Once she conquered her fear, she was able to stand firm, be decisive, do her job well, and regain the respect of her boss, this coworker, and the other members of the team. As a result, the project came to a smooth and successful conclusion, and she was spared several months of unnecessary stress and misery.

Practice Internal Dialogue

Having an internal dialogue is another important tool for conquering fear. By internal dialogue, I'm talking about a conversation with yourself, like a computer checking its internal programming. When you conduct this kind of internal dialogue, you are basically asking yourself:

- What type of person am I?
- What do I believe in?
- What are my standards? Am I willing to compromise them? If so, by how much?

Audit Your Inner Self

Another important question to ask that will help you develop perception and control fear is: What do I want out of this particular situation? A client of mine always asks herself this question when the heat is on at work and she is stressed, angry, or afraid. "All I have to do is to ask myself, 'What do you really want out of this situation? What are your goals?' When I can answer that clearly to myself, I can always put my feelings into perspective and feel much more in control. I can understand that the task at hand is not proving I'm right to everyone, getting the last word, or sometimes even being completely understood. It's about seeing my ultimate goals clearly and knowing I can conquer my fear and move forward if I keep calm and focused."

Taking an internal audit helps you to neutralize fear by creating an intense state of self-awareness. You know what you are capable of because you now understand specifically what you want to achieve—and you have a pretty good idea of how to get there. This is similar to what an athlete does when he goes out onto the field and says to himself, "My opponent is not going to beat me because I know who I am and what I've got." If you can take stock of yourself, telling yourself honestly that you are good at what you do and that you believe in yourself, you can be confident of handling almost any situation.

Visualize Your Outcome

Internal dialogue also involves clearly visualizing your outcome. If before an athlete goes up to the plate he says to himself, "I can't strike out," he's not focusing on the task at hand; he's only thinking about the consequences of possible failure. In other words, he's walking up to the plate with a picture of striking out in his head. And sure enough, nine times out of ten, when he stands up to bat, his body is going to follow the picture of failure he is visualizing in his brain.

But if his self-talk and internal imaging are all about ball place-ment—how he's going to wait for the pitch, how he's going to see the hit, and where he's going to place it—his body is going to do every-thing it can to get him to that point.

I used this technique with my mom recently when she was very sick after a stroke. She wasn't paralyzed, but she couldn't swallow and had to be fed through a tube. The doctors gave her a week to live and told me to start making arrangements for the funeral. Even though they had given up on my mother, I couldn't.

I knew I could only help her if I enabled her to conquer her fear and to visualize a good outcome. She was not able to speak but she could hear me, so I told her what a wonderful mother she'd been to me, and I told her to visualize herself as better. I made sure that everything the doctor and I did for her was focused not just on pro-longing her life for a short time or easing her suffering, but also on her visualizing herself as being well. And, guess what? She got better. As of this writing, she just turned eighty-eight and is able to swallow, eat on her own, and communicate, and she has her full mental facul-ties. The doctor was amazed but told me that he has seen many situa-tions where the power of the mind had directly affected a patient's well-being or longevity.

That's what I call effective internal dialogue coupled with exter-nal performance. Our actions and results always reflect what we think. And ultimately that's the best strategy for managing fear.

6

The Stress Connection

No one can avoid stress. It will be with you, in one form or another, every day of your life—within your working relationships and when you are at home, with friends, on the freeway, in a crowded department store, or watching the evening news. Stressors, great and small, surround us at every turn.

Suppose your alarm clock fails to go off one morning and you discover that you have overslept by half an hour. You shake your husband awake, leap out of bed, take a five-minute shower, skip your makeup, and pull a brush through your hair. Somehow you manage to get both kids dressed, fed, and out the door to the school bus. But you have no time for coffee and your own breakfast, so you start the day hungry and not looking your best. When you get to work, you find out that your secretary is out sick, so you must answer your own phone and deal with tasks that you would normally allocate to him.

Somehow you get through the morning. But when you come up for air, you remember that the Tuesday noon staff meeting has been switched to Monday. Your secretary would normally have reminded you of this, but he isn't there. The quiet lunch you planned is out, so you order a sandwich from the deli and wolf it down in five minutes. All through the meeting you have indigestion.

On your way home you stop at the gas station to fill your nearly empty tank. There is a line of cars waiting and you notice that gas prices have gone up another ten cents per gallon. When you stop by the bank, both of the ATM machines aren't working, so you have to go inside and wait in line to get some cash. When you stop by the grocery store to pick up something for dinner you buy prepackaged, frozen entrées because you are just too tired to cook. Your cell phone rings and it's your husband telling you that he's stuck at the office and won't be home for a couple of hours. When you get home, the nanny is on the phone with her boyfriend and the kids are fighting in the living room. You speak more sharply than you'd like to the nanny, quiet the kids and give them dinner, then eat with your husband when he gets home at nine. You both watch half an hour of television and fall into bed exhausted.

Everyone's life is filled with small stressful episodes like this. None of them, taken individually, will kill you. But over time the effects of constant stress become cumulative, causing your health, well-being, and energy levels to deteriorate. Stress causes wear and tear on the body, keeping you on edge, giving you heartburn and a jumpy stomach, making it difficult for you to sleep soundly at night, unbalancing your hormone levels, elevating your pulse rate, and making you cranky and irritable. It also makes you more susceptible to colds, flu, and more serious types of disease by lowering the efficiency of your immune system. If you factor in lifestyle choices such as being overweight, drinking too much, poor nutritional habits, and not exercising, you are only increasing the long-term effects of stress, both physically and emotionally.

The trick is learning how both to manage stress and to raise your stress threshold. Minor incidents add up over a long time until they do as much damage to your mind and body as one major, traumatic incident. If you don't learn to release stress daily or find a way to make it work for you over the long haul, eventually stress will make you sick or even kill you. It will certainly rob your life of energy, joy, motivation, and fulfillment.

Negative Effects of Stress

Here is a quick overview of some of the negative effects of stress. This list was compiled by Dean Sunseri, M.A., L.P.C. based on findings of experts at the Centers for Disease Control and the National Institute of Occupational Safety and Health.

- Stress is linked to physical and mental health, as well as to decreased willingness to take on new and creative endeavors.
- The job burnout experienced by 25 to 40 percent of U.S. workers is blamed on stress.
- More than ever before, employee stress is being recognized as a major drain on corporate productivity and competitiveness.

- It is predicted that depression, which is only one type of stress reaction, will be the leading occupational disease of the twenty-first century and will be responsible for more days of work lost than any other single factor.
- In the United States $300 billion, or $10,000 per employee, is spent annually on stress-related compensation claims, reduced productivity, absenteeism, health insurance costs, direct medical expenses (nearly 50 percent higher for workers who report stress), and employee turnover.
- The six leading causes of death in the United States—heart disease, cancer, lung ailments, accidents, cirrhosis of the liver, and suicide—are directly related to stress.

What Is Stress?

If stress is so bad for us, why have our bodies developed the stress response in the first place? From an evolutionary standpoint, stress is not only useful but also necessary for our very survival. For the first 200,000 years of humanity's existence, stress was a useful mechanism to get us physically prepared to hunt a wild animal, run for our lives, fight an opponent, or survive a natural disaster such as a flash flood. Greater physical strength from the adrenaline rush, sharper hearing and vision, heightened brain function, and more energy to fight or run were certainly useful.

The catch-22 is that stress is not meant to be a long-term condition of daily life. Our ancestors experienced the heightened physical response of a stress reaction during times of real physical danger, discharged their energy dealing with the problem, and then returned to a physiologically normal state. But in the modern world most of our stress, unless we are getting mugged at knifepoint in a dark alley, is psychological in nature. Therefore it is difficult to make it go away by an immediate action that discharges the stress. When you have twenty hyperactive eight-year-olds over for a birthday party and suddenly the power goes out and you find yourself in the dark, what can you do except light candles, try to avoid burning down the house when a child accidentally knocks one over, and somehow keep them all safe and happy until their parents come to get them in two hours. Yelling at the kids or banging on the kitchen counter with frustration isn't going to solve the problem.

Chemical Changes That Occur during Stress

When you find yourself in a situation that your body perceives as stressful, a number of chemical reactions occur that push certain body systems into higher gear by shutting down or cutting off energy to others.

1. *Stress affects the cardiovascular system.* The first to be affected is the cardiovascular system. In the presence of danger, much of the blood in your outer extremities is shunted to organs that need more oxygen, such as the brain (the decision maker), the heart, and your other vital organs, such as the lungs and the liver. The constricting of the blood supply to your hands, arms, feet, and legs has another role—it decreases your blood loss should you be injured. Your body also increases its production of endorphins and other pain-reducing chemicals so that you won't feel the injury as keenly as you normally would. When these changes happen, your blood pressure rises, your pulse races, and your heart must beat faster and harder to handle the strain. Adrenaline causes glucose and fat to be released from your tissues to give your body a much-needed energy surge in case you must fight or flee.

2. *Some systems shut down.* This enormous surge of energy comes at a price, however. Certain other bodily systems must be shut down somewhat in order to compensate. Your reproductive system, which is normally very energy intensive, is suspended so that its energies can be directed elsewhere. In the short term, this isn't a bad thing, since you would never think about fighting off the cave bear and making love to your mate at the same time. But you can see how living in a constant state of stress would erode your libido over the long term.

3. *How cortisol affects the body.* Another chemical downside following the release of stress hormones is that cortisol accumulates in your body. As the adrenaline rush that released fat and glucose as an energy source subsides, the stress hormone cortisol becomes active, causing insulin to be released to stimulate your appetite so that you can replenish your fat stores. Since most of us don't reach for an apple or a piece of swordfish when we are ravenous, this usually leads to craving a quick carbohydrate snack such as candy, pizza, cookies, ice cream, or high-carbohydrate fast foods. Unfortunately, living with a high level of daily stress causes the body to produce a consistently high level of cortisol, leading to overeating and weight gain, especially in the all-important abdominal area in men.

4. *The immune system is weakened.* One of the more serious effects of stress is the redirecting of energy away from the immune system. A tremendous amount of energy is necessary to operate the complex cells, hormones, and organs that make up this system. Fifteen minutes of danger and a return to normal isn't going to compromise your immune system, but living with constant stress will surely make you more susceptible to illness.

In What Ways Are You Vulnerable to Stress?

One of the first steps toward managing stress is to identify the areas in your life where you are most vulnerable to stress. While no one can eliminate stress from their lives 100 percent, you can always decrease your stress load by modifying the behaviors that are contributing to your stress. The following questionnaire, created by Lyle Miller and Alma Dell Smith of Boston University Medical Center, is designed to help you pinpoint the trouble spots in your life so that you can work on them. Nearly all of the questions listed refer to situations and behaviors over which you have a great deal of control. If you score higher than 3 on any item, try to modify that behavior. Try first to modify those behaviors that seem easiest for you to change and work your way up to the ones you perceive as difficult.

Score each item from 1 (always) to 5 (never), according to how often the statement accurately describes your behaviors. Be sure to mark each item, even if it does not apply to you. For example, if you do not smoke, circle 1 for that question. To figure your score, add up all the numbers and subtract 20. A score below 10 indicates a high resistance to stress. A score over 30 indicates a moderate vulnerability to stress. If your score is over 50, you have a serious vulnerability to stress.

How Vulnerable Are You to Stress?

	Always	Some-times	Never
	1	2 3 4	5
1. I eat at least one hot, balanced meal per day.	☐	☐☐☐	☐
2. I get 7 to 8 hours sleep at least 4 nights a week.	☐	☐☐☐	☐
3. I give and receive affection regularly.	☐	☐☐☐	☐
4. I have at least one relative within 50 miles upon whom I can rely.	☐	☐☐☐	☐

	Always	Some- times	Never
	1	2 3 4	5

5. I exercise to the point of perspiration at least twice a week. ☐ ☐☐☐ ☐

6. I limit myself to less than half a pack of cigarettes a day. ☐ ☐☐☐ ☐

7. I have fewer than five alcoholic drinks a week. ☐ ☐☐☐ ☐

8. I am the appropriate weight for my height. ☐ ☐☐☐ ☐

9. I have an income adequate to meet basic expenses. ☐ ☐☐☐ ☐

10. I get strength from my religious beliefs. ☐ ☐☐☐ ☐

11. I regularly attend club or social activities. ☐ ☐☐☐ ☐

12. I have a network of friends and acquaintances. ☐ ☐☐☐ ☐

13. I have one or more friends to confide in about personal matters. ☐ ☐☐☐ ☐

14. I am in good health (including eyesight, hearing, and teeth). ☐ ☐☐☐ ☐

15. I am able to speak openly about my feelings when I am angry. ☐ ☐☐☐ ☐

16. I have regular conversations with the people with whom I live about domestic problems— for example, chores and money. ☐ ☐☐☐ ☐

17. I do something for fun at least once a week. ☐ ☐☐☐ ☐

18. I am able to organize my time effectively. ☐ ☐☐☐ ☐

19. I drink fewer than three cups of coffee (or other caffeine-rich drinks) a day. ☐ ☐☐☐ ☐

20. I take some quiet time for myself during the day. ☐ ☐☐☐ ☐

Evaluate Your Stress Behaviors

I also find this brief stress questionnaire by Dean Sunseri to be quite helpful in identifying areas of stress in your life. Answering yes to any of these behaviors is a sure indication that a significant amount of stress has accumulated in your life.

A Quick Stress Evaluation

	Yes	No

1. Do you have difficulty sleeping because you are constantly thinking about a future event or completing a certain task? ☐ ☐

	Yes	No
2. Have your eating habits changed in an unhealthy way because your schedule is too busy?	☐	☐
3. Is your schedule so busy that you don't have time for leisure or fun activities?	☐	☐
4. Do you have tightness or stiffness in your shoulder or stomach area?	☐	☐
5. Do you have a difficult time slowing down and function as if you are run by a motor?	☐	☐
6. Is your level of anxiety higher than normal?	☐	☐

The Rahe Life Stress Scale

The well-known Rahe Life Stress Scale, developed by Dr. Thomas Holmes, M.D., and Richard H. Rahe, M.D., two researchers at the University of Washington School of Medicine in Seattle, actually assigns a number to a stressful event, based on Holmes's and Rahe's years of research regarding the connection between stress and health. For example, the death of a spouse is 119 points, pregnancy is 67, divorce is 96, changing jobs is 51, and having sexual difficulties is 44. Even events that you might think of as being positive have an impact on your stress load. Marriage is 50 points, a major increase in income is 38 points, a vacation is 24, and the birth of a grandchild is 43. According to Holmes and Rahe, if you score below 200, you have a low risk of illness. Between 201 and 300, your chances of getting sick are moderate. A score between 301 and 450 increases your odds considerably, and a score greater than 450 puts you at imminent risk. If you wish to take this test, you can access it on the Internet at Dr. Rahe's Web site, www.hapi-health.com.

Keep in mind, however, that your score is not an absolute indicator of your actual risk for disease. According to Janelle M. Barlow, Ph.D., author of *The Stress Manager,* a study conducted by Dr. Suzanne Kobassa at the University of Chicago showed that certain individuals who had high stress scores actually enjoyed fairly good health. These individuals, whom Dr. Kobassa called the "hardy executives," all had the following characteristics:

- An internal sense of control
- Action oriented
- High levels of self-esteem
- A life plan with established priorities

Dan: The Hardy Executive

I have a client named Dan who is a good example of the hardy executive. Dan, a forty-year-old vice president of a major bank, often does not get home until eight-thirty at night and, during certain times of the year, works seven days a week. His demanding workload, which used to be parceled out between two other employees, carries a high level of stress and responsibility. If he took the Rahe Life Stress Scale, he would likely score relatively high.

Yet Dan, thanks to my program, is fit, slender, and in good health. He has a positive self-image, exercises regularly with weights, is very good at problem solving, is great with people, and is very intelligent. He and his wife have almost paid off their home, have planned well for their retirement (which they will both take early), have made wise investments, and have even provided for the college education of their six-year-old daughter. Their lives are well organized, and they both take time off for pleasure, such as playing golf and taking family vacations.

Most of us, however, have not yet mastered the art of being a hardy executive. We need to develop special skills to manage our stress and increase our stress threshold before it makes us emotionally upset and then physically ill.

Stress and Nutrition

In a healthy person who is fasting or starving, 90 percent of their calories will come from fat stores and only 10 percent from protein. When a person is undergoing significant and continual stress, even if they are not injured or sick, only 70 percent of their calories will come from fat stores, and 30 percent will come from lean protein. The breakdown of protein for fuel comes as a direct response to the body's greater need for glucose during times of stress. Glucose comes from amino acids taken from lean muscle mass that are then converted to alanine, and then to glucose to be dispersed to all of the tissues as an emergency energy supply. After surgery, a person's metabolic rate increases 20 percent, and after a severe burn 100 percent. A wound, infection, or traumatic injury falls between these two extremes with a 50 percent increase.

You can see, then, that following a well-balanced and nutritional food program such as the one I will present in chapter 10 becomes even more crucial when you are undergoing the effects of illness or long-term stress. This can be seen in the story of a client of mine who had difficulty healing following an automobile accident.

Bronwen totaled her brand-new car on the freeway 450 miles from home on her way to a health conference. Her airbag saved her life, and she had no serious injuries other than severe bruising of her arms and chest. But the trauma of arranging for her now undriveable car to be repaired so far from home; coordinating towing costs and repairs with a branch office of her insurance company; and getting herself back home took its toll on her energy reserves. Added to this was the stress of getting her house fumigated for termites a week after she returned. There was no way she could cancel or reschedule this appointment. So in her physically and emotionally weakened state, she was forced to pack up and prepare the house, which added to her stress load.

While she was moving some boxes, her cat became startled and scratched her leg. Bronwen, who is physically fit, slender, and enjoys excellent health, thought nothing of this. She usually doesn't even wash out a cat scratch because she heals so well. However, this small scratch quickly became so infected that she could hardly walk on her leg and had to take antibiotics. Eventually, after she could return to her home, rest, and get her routine back to normal, her infected leg and bruises from the car accident healed. But she was in a state of severe stress and great pain during the entire time she had to pack her house, stay at a friend's home during the fumigation, and unpack upon her return.

What is significant about Bronwen's story is not only the burden that stress put upon her body's normal ability to heal, but also her lack of good nutritional habits during this time. Because she was so busy and so stressed, Bronwen sometimes neglected to eat during these events. While the regular food program my nutritionist had designed for her was sufficient to keep her body working properly under normal conditions of stress and metabolic activity, it was not sufficient to help her heal during a two-week period of severe physical and emotional stress. Bronwen ate less, not more, and felt worse and worse.

When she finally phoned me for help, I told her how important it was for her to follow her nutrition program to the letter, eating three well-balanced meals each day and two snacks. I also encouraged her to increase the amount of protein in her daily diet to 100 grams per day until her body healed, since protein is what repairs muscle tissue and injury, and to make sure that she took all her supplements faithfully. After a few days, Bronwen began feeling much better physically and less stressed.

This story and what we have already seen about how chronic stress weakens the immune system illustrate why an important part of any stress management program is proper nutrition. Your body simply will not be able to bear up under the effects of stress without appropriate fuel.

Stress, High Blood Pressure, and Heart Disease

As we have seen, any time you face a stressful situation, your body rushes blood to your brain and organ systems. This is not a problem over the short term, but constant stress can lead to hypertension (high blood pressure) and heart disease. For example, being downsized from your job will probably create additional stresses as you rebalance your finances, your relationship with your spouse, and your self-esteem while hunting for a new job. Your tension and blood pressure levels will be quite high for weeks or even months until you get things sorted out again. This increased hypertension could cause a blood vessel to rupture, causing a heart attack.

Beta-blockers are medications used to lower blood pressure and are essentially designed to prevent the body from producing stress-related chemicals. But ultimately the body will continue to elevate those chemicals when under prolonged stress, no matter how many blood pressure medications you are using. The only cure for hypertension is stress management and instituting lifestyle changes such as weight loss and proper nutrition.

The NFL Combine is a yearly event that takes place in the Indianapolis Hoosier Dome where scouts and coaches from each of the major teams gather to look over and audition new prospective talent for their teams in preparation for the upcoming NFL draft. These players are usually college seniors in their early twenties.

One year a young man named Greg came to see me with a knee injury. Greg weighed 340 pounds, had a waist measurement of 50 inches, and was a standout player at a major university. While the nurse was taking his history, I said, "Do you mind taking his blood pressure?" Sitting down, Greg's pressure was 140 over 85. According to the latest figures, anything over the diastolic figure 85 represents borderline risk. While a systolic number of 140 isn't bad, it's better to keep that figure in the 130s.

I asked the technician to take Greg's pressure again while he was standing. When Greg stood up, his pressure went up to 145 over 90. This was a 23-year-old young man! I asked his mother, who was sitting in the room, if there was any history of hypertension in the family. As it turned out, Greg's uncle died from a stroke.

High blood pressure in someone as young as Greg is more widespread than you would think. A recent study of freshmen coming into college football programs found that 24 percent had abnormal blood lipids. Some of these students had high blood pressure as well. I have been encountering hypertension more and more in the promising college athletes who take part in my performance enhancement programs. The lifestyle profiles of these young men are very similar. They eat a lot of fast foods with high fat and salt content, are carrying too much weight, and have a high percentage of body fat. And they don't have a clue that they have high blood pressure. Everyone perceives them as being big strong football players. Chances are they would never even know they had hypertension unless they were tested for it.

Take responsibility for your health and take it early in life.

The greater flow of blood to your cranial vessels caused by the body's stress response increases the pressure inside those vessels. The longer one's stress levels continue to remain high on a daily basis, the greater the vulnerability to stroke. To make matters worse, the brain responds to higher levels of blood pressure by thickening its blood vessels. This results in pressure on nearby nerves, causing headaches and loss of the blood vessels' flexibility, making them more liable to rupture during extreme surges of blood, causing stroke.

Since the stress response elevates chemicals that increase the amount of fat (an energy source) in your blood stream, long-term stress also makes you more vulnerable to developing high cholesterol. High blood pressure, if allowed to continue unchecked, will exacerbate this process, eventually causing small tears within the walls of your arteries that will collect the LDL (bad cholesterol fats) racing through your bloodstream due to stress elevation. The very hormones that cause stress also destroy HDL, the good cholesterol that keeps your blood vessels clear by counteracting the negative effects of too much LDL.

If you lead a stress-filled life, the elevated blood sugar levels in your body will eventually make you vulnerable to type 2 diabetes, the fourth leading cause of death in the United States. During short-term stress, you would normally burn off the increase in glucose production, but not if you live with constant worry and anxiety. Long-term stress will leave you with permanently elevated blood sugar.

Stress Contributes to Some Cancers

While the relationship between stress and cancer has not been definitely proven, enough information has been gathered to cause researchers to continue to explore the question. For example, the National Cancer Institute reports that some studies of women with breast cancer have shown significantly higher rates of occurrence of this disease among women who have experienced traumatic life events and stress within several years of their diagnosis. These factors include death of a spouse, social isolation, and other psychological factors.

Studies are also under way to explore the effects of stress on the immune response of women already diagnosed with cancer to see if stress reduction can slow the progression of the cancer. One major study conducted by Ohio State University and published in the *Journal of the National Cancer Institute* involved high-stress and low-stress women following surgery for stage II and stage III breast cancer. The researchers found that the women who reported high levels of personal stress had significantly lower blood levels of three important immune factors. The first two were the NK cells, which play a large role in the immune system's search for tumors and virally infected cells, and T-lymphocytes, also known as white blood cells. When the researchers exposed the NK cells within the bloodstream of the high-stress women to extra amounts of gamma interferon, a compound that naturally enhances NK cell activity and the replication of viruses, they found a third significantly lowered immune response. The more stress a woman reported, the less effect the gamma interferon had on her NK cells.

Stress and Inflammatory Bowel Diseases

There have been several studies about the effects of stress on people suffering from inflammatory bowel diseases such as Crohn's disease and ulcerative colitis. (Inflammatory bowel disease is a condition in which a person's immune system attacks its own body.) A recent article in *Nature Medicine* quoted Dr. Stephen Collins, chief of gastroenterology at McMaster University in Hamilton, Ontario as saying, "[Stress] is, in my opinion, a very common reason for flare-ups of the disease. . . . There is indeed a causal link between stress and relapse, and this should motivate [patients] to address coping with stress in their lives." Among the evidence that Dr. Collins and his colleagues observed in their study was the effects of stress on the mucous membranes of the colon, making them more porous and more susceptible to being attacked by the individual's own immune system.

I have a client called Ann, whom I have successfully helped to manage her ulcerative colitis for eight years. Stress management—along with appropriate nutrition and exercise—has been instrumental in helping her keep her condition under control. When Ann's husband, an officer in the Coast Guard, was arrested and imprisoned while trying to file conscientious objector status during the Gulf War after his unit had been called up, Ann's colitis flared up to such a degree that she went down to eighty-six pounds and almost died. That was when she came to me and we began an intensive study of how nutrition and stress management could alleviate symptoms of her disease. Ann, who has a Ph.D. in psychotherapy, now uses stress management as part of her therapeutic approach when working with her clients.

Stress Can Cause Brain Damage and Memory Loss

One of the body's responses to stress is a heightened mental state and the ability to think on your feet. While this sounds wonderful, the downside is that the chemical that causes this mental alertness, cortisol, also kills brain cells. According to Dr. Robert Sapolsky, a Stanford University biologist who has extensively researched the physical effects of stress, the cells that are most vulnerable to destruction are the ones located in the hippocampus, the part of the brain responsible for memory. The hippocampus is also the area that deteriorates when patients contract Alzheimer's disease and other memory disorders. This research seems to point to the idea that prolonged stress could be directly related to memory problems and other cognitive disorders.

Now that we've seen the toll that stress takes on the body and the emotions, let's look at several strategies for managing stress.

7

Master Stress Management for Maximum Performance

As strange as it may sound, many people are not even aware of the moment when they cross their stress threshold. For some, stress has become such a natural state that they are used to operating within a state of high arousal. Indeed, some individuals actually become so addicted to stress that they cannot summon creative energies or make their deadlines without the additional push that stress gives them. We've all seen this type of personality in people with high-pressure jobs: the attorney, the emergency room doctor, the stockbroker, the writer on a deadline, the working mom, the high-powered CEO. Then there are those who rush through life overscheduling their time, taking on more and more, leaving things to the last minute, working twelve hours a day, telling themselves that they can do it all. For all of these individuals, stress has become almost like a drug.

Manage Your Stress Threshold

I recently helped a client name Stephanie who deals with the high-pressure world of contract law to manage her stress threshold. Contract law involves getting both sides to agree to a certain level of compromise. I have noticed that women tend to have a different relationship to stress than men do. They tend to take stress into themselves and then let it back out, while a little remains behind. Stephanie would arbitrate with each side, internalize their stress, then let it back out, each time inadvertently leaving a little bit more behind in her body.

Stephanie's body reacted to this accumulation of stress by developing immune dysfunction. She became much more susceptible to colds and flus, developed painful rashes almost like shingles, and suffered from migraines. She also developed cytomegalovirus, a type of chronic fatigue syndrome that only presents when a person crosses his stress threshold.

I created a three-part program to help Stephanie release her accumulated stress:

- I put her on my Pro Circuit Exercise Program (see chapter 13) to allow her to recharge herself. By training her at her appropriate target heart rate, we conditioned her body to learn how to automatically deal with and release stress.
- I recommended that she take a course in transcendental meditation and, before every arbitration session, do a ten-minute meditation, relaxing and repeating the mantra *om* to lower her resting heart rate. I also taught her how to release stress during sessions with clients by putting her hand under the table, making a fist, and repeating to herself, "Release."
- I instructed her to stabilize her blood sugar by always eating breakfast before an arbitration and encouraged her to keep on hand a supply of low-carbohydrate, high-protein energy bars to eat on breaks so that she could stabilize her blood sugar every three hours.

On this program, Stephanie transformed herself from a participant to a spectator and was able to keep the stress in the room where it belonged, in someone else's body, not hers.

How Much Stress Is Too Much?

Stress is an unavoidable part of life. Minimizing and managing stress is a learned art. The point at which one crosses the stress threshold into harmful stress is different for every person. A certain amount of stress can be a healthy catalyst toward doing your best and surpassing your limitations. Too much stress can be a ticket for early death from burnout, heart attack, stroke, type 2 diabetes, emotional instability, irritability, and depression.

The first step toward managing stress is to become more aware of your daily states of arousal and relaxation and to pay attention to how they make you feel. Your ultimate mastery in the battle of stress management will be for you to find ways consciously to deactivate the flight-or-fight response when it does not serve you, as well as activate the relaxation response at will.

Biofeedback: Feel the Difference between Arousal and Relaxation

In her book *The High Performance Mind: Mastering Brainwaves for Insight, Healing, and Creativity,* Anna Wise offers some simple exercises to help you become aware of the difference between feeling aroused, ready to fight or to flee, and feeling relaxed and in control of the situation.

When a person experiences feelings of worry, excitement, fear, anger, exhilaration, nervousness, panic, increased heart rate, faster breathing, and/or anxiety, the sympathetic nervous system is activated. When a person feels a sense of relaxation, tranquility, calmness, serenity, lightness, centeredness, clarity and/or a feeling of being in control, the parasympathetic system is activated.

Wise suggests that you can achieve greater awareness of when you are stressed and when you are relaxed by performing the following exercises and observing your biofeedback—how your body feels.

- Hyperventilate by breathing heavily for a few seconds. (Please be careful not to overdo it. If you start to feel faint, stop immediately.)

  [Stop. Close your eyes. Notice what your body feels like. Make a mental note of all the sensations.]

- Run in place for a minute or two.
- Think about something very upsetting.
- Think about something very exciting.

After each one of these, stop and notice what is happening inside of your body.

The physical state of arousal you are in while doing these exercises will be similar to how your body responds when exposed to stress.

Next notice how your body feels when completely relaxed:

Close your eyes and exhale deeply. Let your shoulders drop. Rotate your head gently and loosely until you find a comfortable balanced position for your head, neck, and shoulders. Let your jaw relax and hang loose. Relax your lips, tongue, and throat. Exhale deeply again and let go. Continue to breathe easily, slowly, evenly, and deeply for one or two minutes.

Stop. Notice what your body feels like. Make a mental note of all of the sensations. Compare these to the sensations you noted when you did the arousal exercises.

Wise goes on to explain, "Arousal is not inherently better than relaxation, or vice versa. Both states are important *at certain times*. What is optimum is *to be able to choose the level of relaxation or arousal that you want and to be able to produce that at will*."

Negative Effects of On-the-Job Stress

For many of us, most of our stress is encountered in the workplace because we spend so much time there. A lot depends on our ability to financially support ourselves and our families and to achieve success in the eyes of the world. Therefore it is important to develop tools for managing on-the-job stress.

According to Dean Sunseri, individuals who do not manage their work-related stress have a higher level of absenteeism, decreased work performance, and emotional instability at their jobs. In their personal lives, this inability to manage stress leads to relationship problems, emotional isolation, substance abuse, verbal/physical violence, and increased high-risk behaviors such as alcoholism.

A recent study by Drs. Nicole A. Roberts and Robert W. Levenson of U.C. Berkeley, published in the *Journal of Marriage and Family*, shows that high levels of on-the-job stress seem to play a significant role in marital problems and could potentially lead to divorce if the stress isn't acknowledged and managed. "These influences of job stress were found regardless of couples' marital satisfaction, husbands' work shift, and couples' parenthood status," the authors wrote. They went on to suggest that when job stress levels become highest, couples should make an extra effort to be attuned to themselves so that they could find ways to handle their stress in a constructive manner. "This may include employing stress management techniques, making an effort to infuse positive emotions into marital conversations, and finding ways to talk about job stress rather than avoiding it."

This is often easier said than done. According to a recent article in the New Orleans *Times-Picayune,* job stress can sneak up on you so gradually that you don't even realize it. Many employees entering the workforce are young and single with ample time for leisure activities, exercise, rest, and sports. As they grow older, marry, have children, and acquire a mortgage and other major responsibilities, their stress load will build and their productivity levels drop. Add to this the fact that many companies lay off employees during times of economic recession, burdening those who remain with an increased workload and even greater stress.

Recently I saw a dramatic example of this when a shipping company called me to inquire about my corporate program. Their top salesperson, a middle-aged man named Arnold, had serious physical problems. Arnold was 400 pounds, had a fifty-two-inch waist, and had a blood sugar level of 126, which made him diabetic. Arnold hadn't been this heavy or this sick when he first went to work for them. But the stresses of his workload and the amount of constant traveling he had to do had brought him to this point. Arnold was a prime candidate to drop dead of a heart attack. And if he had, his company would have been in serious trouble. Fortunately, Arnold is thrilled with the program and has already lost twenty-five pounds.

Dee Edington, director of Michigan's Health Management Research Center, has spent twenty-five years researching how major corporations have saved literally millions of dollars in health care costs by offering services to their employees such as wellness programs, on-site gyms and fitness programs, and health newsletters. What Edington stresses, however, is that companies should not focus on just those employees whose stress loads and health needs are the greatest. There are tremendous long-term benefits in retaining relatively healthy employees who eat right, exercise regularly, and manage their stress healthfully. "It is much easier to help a low-risk person remain low-risk than to try to change a high-risk person to low-risk," Edington says.

Unfortunately, most corporations do not take responsibility for their employees' health. Even if you are fairly healthy, you cannot count on your workplace to take responsibility to help you maintain your health and emotional well-being. Ultimately, that responsibility falls squarely on your shoulders.

In this fast-paced, stress-filled world, the only answer is to develop your own stress management skills. I have found the following stress management techniques to be tremendously effective. I suggest that you experiment with one or a combination of these until you find what works best for you.

Eight Steps for Controlling Stress at the Office

It would be wonderful if all corporations provided their employees with meditation rooms and built mandatory recovery breaks into everyone's busy schedule. In fact, studies have shown that these kinds of activities actually increase productivity. Since that day is still far in the future, Anna Wise offers eight meditation exercises one can practice in the office to deactivate the stress response and become more relaxed, creative, and balanced during the workday. I have included that list here.

1. **Make ample use of one-minute meditations.** Obviously, this will be easier if you are working in a private space than if you are sharing an office. These include the following:
   - Sit in a relaxed posture and breathe deeply, in and out, for one minute.
   - Focus on relaxing your tongue and jaw for one minute.
   - Intentionally slow your breathing for one minute.
   - Sitting comfortably with your eyes gently open, focus your awareness on a spot outside of yourself for one minute.
   - Sitting comfortably with your eyes closed, focus your awareness on a particular location *inside* yourself, such as your heart, your third eye, or your navel.
   - Imagine a friend's face smiling at you.
   - Imagine receiving a warm hug from an old friend.
2. **Breathe!** The most calming action you can take when faced with stress is to consciously focus on slowing your rate of breathing. For example, while you are listening to problems or complaints from a superior, you can at the same time be aware of your rhythmical and slow breathing and your relaxed heart rate. This not only helps to keep you calm, but gives you the detachment that helps provide proper perspective when dealing with crisis.

3. When faced with stressful situations **make a complete energy circuit in your body**. Sit with the palms of your hands together or—just as effective—the tips of the thumb pads and middle fingers touching one another. This helps contain the flow of energy within your body and maintain centeredness and balance.

4. **Sit with your spine straight and relaxed**, and your legs uncrossed. This also unblocks energy, which can then be called upon for use.

5. **Sensualize!** If you are facing a very difficult encounter or situation, take a few minutes to be by yourself before it begins. Using all of your senses, imagine the situation occurring in the most successful and healthy way possible. Imagine your own actions and reactions to be calm, strong, creative, and appropriate.

6. **Use ordinary activity as a meditation practice.** For example, when you are going to the watercooler for a drink, take the opportunity to be awake and aware. Be aware of each move as you make it and be very present in the actual act—not drawn back into the past or forward into the future. Be sensually aware of the smells, tastes, sights, sounds, textures, and kinesthesia of the situation. Savor every second of the experience, while remaining in the present.

7. **Look for allies among your coworkers.** You might be surprised to find other meditators more prevalent than you thought. There is support in numbers—if meditation becomes an acceptable and even pleasantly anticipated topic of conversation, your practices will be supported and you will feel freer to practice more frequently and more openly.

8. **Support others** in the need for and value of contemplative time.

Attitude Breathing

Another resource I have found helpful are the techniques developed by Doc Childre, founder of the Institute of HeartMath. The institute's work has resulted in over a decade of leading edge research on the connection between the mind, body, and emotions. Many of their studies have been published in leading peer review journals and led to a number of powerful techniques to help neutralize stress in the moment. Below is one technique called Attitude Breathing that Doc recommends for starting your day from a point of balance. You can use this in any situation when stress is closing in on you.

Attitude Breathing: Sometimes it can be hard to stop negative thoughts or draining moods. At these times, using the Attitude Breathing tool helps you anchor your inner power and bring your thoughts and emotions back into balance. Practicing Attitude Breathing is like soaking your uncomfortable feelings in a comforting bath. It takes the "fire" out of negative thoughts and emotions so they have less fuel and power.

To prepare to use this tool, take a moment to build an attitude of appreciation for someone or something and imagine you are breathing that feeling of appreciation through your heart for two or three breaths. Next, follow these three steps:

Step 1. Shift your attention to your heart and solar plexus/stomach area.

Step 2. Ask yourself, "What would be a better attitude for me to maintain in this situation?" Then, set up an inner attitude, like "Stay calm," "Stay neutral in this situation," "Don't judge before you know the facts," "Make peace with this," or decide what attitude is appropriate for your situation.

Step 3. Next gently and sincerely pretend to breathe the new attitude you want in through the heart. Then breathe it out through the solar plexus and stomach to anchor it. Do this for a while until you feel the new attitude has set in.

Attitude Breathing is an easy and useful tool you can use in a wide variety of situations. Here are some of them:

- When you wake up in the morning: Thoughts and emotions like anxiety, worry, sadness, hurt, or anger can often try to creep in as soon as you wake up in the morning, sometimes before you even get out of bed. Practice Attitude Breathing within the first 30 minutes to an hour after you awaken, as you remember it during your preparations for the day. You can do it while in the shower, getting dressed for work, or during your commute. The reason for doing this is that those negative thoughts and attitudes you wake up with can quickly increase in momentum if you don't neutralize and replace them with attitudes that are not self-draining. Choose the thoughts and attitudes that would benefit your day and breathe them in through the heart and out through the solar plexus and abdomen area. The outward breath through the solar plexus anchors the attitude. Remember that you don't have to stop regular activities to use the Attitude Breathing tool.

- Releasing tension or anxiety: A buildup of tension is an indicator of being out of balance emotionally. Some of us accumulate tension in the area of the chest. We may experience shortness of breath, heart palpitations, or irregular heartbeats. Others experience tension as a headache or a knot in the stomach, back, neck, or shoulders. Use Attitude Breathing to help release tension in any part of the body. As you do this, ask yourself, "What would be a more balanced feeling or approach to what I'm doing?" Once you feel more emotionally balanced, then pretend to breathe the feeling of balance through the area of tension. You'll start to feel the tension release as more of your balanced heart energy moves through that area.
- Stopping emotional reactivity: During stressful times, many people are experiencing more negative emotions, such as anxiety, fear, uncertainty, grief, and anger. This can make us more edgy and irritable and sometimes cause us to react strongly to others before we think twice about it. When you feel yourself beginning to react emotionally to someone or something, use Attitude Breathing to take the excess negative emotion out of your reaction. Anchoring your energy in your heart and solar plexus will help you stay centered and see calmly and clearly how best to respond.

You can learn more about HeartMath's research and their techniques at their Web site: www.heartmath.com.

Recite Calming Prayers and Mantras

A recent study published in the *British Medical Journal* reported that age-old practices such as repeating the Catholic prayer Hail Mary or a mantra decreased stress by regulating the breathing. Other studies bear this out, such as one conducted at the School of Internal Medicine at the University of Pavia in Italy, which found that slow rhythmic breathing—about six breaths per minute—synchronizes internal heart-lung rhythms and improves blood oxygen levels and cardiovascular responsiveness.

Reciting familiar prayers and mantras was found to have exactly that effect upon the body of test subjects.

Dr. Herbert Benson, president of the Mind/Body Medical Institute and associate professor of medicine at Harvard Medical School, calls the physiological state achieved during prayer and meditation the "relaxation response," since it reduces metabolism, blood pressure, and heart rate. It also induces slow and rhythmic brain waves. Benson states that this state can be deepened further if the person reciting the prayer or mantra attributes some kind of spiritual significance to these phrases. It is easy to understand why monasteries are such places of peace, stillness, and repose.

Practice Detachment

Worry, anxiety, behaving compulsively, and being in an unhealthy relationship with a friend, significant other, or coworker are all forms of attachment that cause stress.

It is not easy to stop worrying about the present and the future, to cease feeling obligated to those to whom we really aren't obligated, and to separate yourself from tasks and responsibilities that really belong to others. The first step toward detachment is to identify the things in your life that do not belong there. This can be done by sitting down and making a list with two headings: "My Life and Responsibilities" and "Other People's Lives and Responsibilities." Once you have identified which things in life you are not responsible for, you can start consciously disassociating yourself from them one by one.

Many of us do not realize how addicted we have become to solving other people's problems and helping them to see how much easier, less stressed, and efficient their lives would be if only they would do things *our way*. In his book *Growing Yourself Back Up: Understanding Emotional Regression*, psychotherapist and workshop leader John Lee shows readers that it is arrogant and self-defeating for us to assume that we can solve other people's problems for them. It uses up our energy reserves, causes us stress, and usually doesn't help anyone anyway.

One of the most constructive things we can do for others—be they friends, family, or coworkers—is to allow them to make their own decisions, their own choices, their own mistakes, and to experience their own victories. How else can we expect them to learn except by doing for themselves? We can't control the amount of stress in other people's lives, but we can surely greatly reduce our own by not assuming responsibility for the stress of others.

Cultivate Healthy and Loving Relationships

While codependence serves no one, working to create healthy and emotionally stable relationships in our lives does much to keep our stress levels low. In their book *Feeling Good Is Good for You: How Pleasure Can Boost Your Immune System and Lengthen Your Life,* Drs. Carl Charnetski and Francis Brennan point out that we are at our happiest and healthiest when we have loving people in our lives. Studies have shown that chronically lonely people have greater instances of illness, lower levels of life satisfaction, and even earlier death rates than people who have significant others in their lives. The authors write: "Do you have people to lean on, people to talk to you, people to tell you that, despite your doubts, everything will work out? That's emotional support, and it can come from anyone—a lover, parents, other family members, friends, neighbors, acquaintances at the gym or country club, members of a church group, coworkers, the bowling league, even seemingly impersonal cyber-friends on the internet."

Although the research is still in its infancy a growing number of studies have shown that people who are in good marriages or love relationships live longer. These individuals have stronger immune systems, have fewer hospital stays and less serious diagnosis upon admission, are less likely to die in the hospital, and are less likely to be placed in nursing homes upon discharge. Even cancer does not seem to progress as rapidly in their bodies.

On the other hand, getting out of a bad marriage or relationship has been shown to be one of the best methods for managing stress and improving your overall health and immune function. The stress of a toxic relationship can make you physically sick.

Women: Stress Management through Bonding

For the last five decades 90 percent of all stress research has used men as subjects, but a recent landmark study on women and stress conducted at UCLA shows surprising differences between how the two genders respond to stress. While men usually respond with the classic "fight or flight" behavior, women more often manage stress by seeking out bonding activities.

Dr. Laura Cousino Klein, one of the study's authors, says that the mechanism behind this response is the release of the hormone oxytocin. While the large amounts of testosterone produced in men during stress tends to counteract this hormone, estrogen enhances its effect. Oxytocin buffers the fight-or-flight response in women and encourages them to tend children and bond with other women instead. These "tending or befriending" behaviors cause the body to release more oxytocin, producing a further calming affect.

This new stress research may help to shed light on why women so consistently outlive men. Study after study has shown that developing close social ties reduces a person's risk of disease by lowering blood pressure, heart rate, and cholesterol. In fact, the famous Nurses' Health Study from Harvard Medical School found that the more friends a woman had, the more likely she was to lead a joyful life and the less likely to develop physical problems and impairments.

If you are a woman in the business world, just be aware that one of your most powerful tools for managing stress is the strength and friendship of other women.

Bishop Morton: Treat Your Body Like a Temple

Consistent exercise is one of the most important lifestyle changes that can help in the management of stress. In fact, the physical and emotional benefits of exercise can actually help you to increase your stress threshold to a greater degree.

Just as stress weakens the body, so exercise strengthens it, giving you more energy, greater emotional stability, and a higher level of health. It also gives your body a chance to reduce the fight-or-flight chemicals that have been collecting in your bloodstream during the course of a stressful day. Exercise is key to achieving a greater level of performance and creativity in your life and profession. Regular exercise is especially important for those individuals who cannot avoid high levels of daily stress.

One of my clients, Dr. Paul Morton, presiding bishop of the Full Gospel Baptist Church Fellowship, is a prime example. He joined my program because he felt overwhelmed with the stress of his demanding position. Bishop Morton has one of the largest followings in the country. He started out with one church, but now his churches have moved into several surrounding states. Although the bishop is a quiet man when you speak with him privately, in his public persona, he's a man who captures your attention, throwing energy out right and left. His sermons are filled with energy and dramatic power—and he often gives more than one a day because they are being videotaped.

Bishop Morton told me that he had spent a lifetime teaching and preaching about how to balance things. But while he was an expert when it came to spiritual issues, he didn't know very much about how to balance the physical side of life. "Sometimes," he said, "even ministers and bishops can overwork themselves. And it is important that you have a plan to counteract this. I found that the right kind of exercise relieves your mind of a lot of stress, that and learning how to eat right."

Doing my Pro Circuit Exercise Program, which I describe in chapter 13, was liberating for the bishop. Regular exercise gave him a focus for his mind, an escape from stress, and a renewed sense of peace, energy, and physical well-being that he hadn't felt in a long time. Learning how to eat nutritionally also helped the bishop reduce his stress load. Before, he had skipped breakfast, eaten sporadically, and eaten all the wrong kinds of foods, which left him dealing with a stressful schedule without proper fueling. Since the bishop was constantly in the public eye, he also had to deal with his weight gain and the stress of his constant attempts to diet. "I was teaching, from the spiritual end, that your body is the temple of God. So many times we think about drugs and alcohol and your body. But we really have to be careful about what we eat. I was always suffering, going up and down, up and down with my weight. That would wear me down and depress me."

When I asked the bishop how long it took him to experience results from the Pro Circuit Program, he told me that he began feeling more energized, less stressed, and less exhausted within two days, but that it took about thirty days for him to see the full benefits. These included noticeable weight loss, satisfaction with his appearance, better performance, a lack of depression, greater emotional evenness, and an increased ability to cope with the demands of his busy schedule without feeling overwhelmed with stress.

Raise the Bar of Your Performance

I often ask my clients to visualize life as a series of high-jump bars. In many situations we can control how high the bar will be, setting it at a level we know we can handle. But situations constantly arise when we are forced to "raise the bar." At such times, when we are being asked to perform above our perceived capabilities, our stress levels rise. The boss at work might challenge us with an especially difficult project. Our significant other might suddenly demand a greater level of investment in our marriage or love relationship. The bar is raised when we have our first child, when money gets tight and we must come up with creative solutions to juggle our finances, when we want to buy our first home or a bigger home. Sometimes we raise the bar ourselves when we demand more of ourselves creatively, and we want to achieve greater accomplishments than we ever have before.

Everyone expects athletes to continually meet—and even surpass—their past performance levels. That's why athletes require the support of performance enhancement specialists such as myself who train them for peak performance and longevity. No athlete would ever go onto the field without training for the season. Nor would they be able to deal with the cumulative effects of injury and physical stress without a solid nutrition and exercise program to help them stay balanced and continue to get the most they can from the assets they have.

Everyone who has a demanding job or lifestyle—and who doesn't?—needs to begin thinking of himself or herself as a different type of athlete, one that is in training for the game of life. No high jumper would try to clear the bar while carrying around burdens such as excessive weight, poor health, smoking and alcohol abuse, improper nutrition, high cholesterol, or high blood sugar. All of these factors put the body under terrific strain.

Just as boxers train themselves to endure greater and greater levels of stress and physical exertion in the ring, so you can use the tools in this chapter to increase your own stress threshold. To avoid the physical and emotional effects of debilitating stress, you must learn to take your nutrition, exercise program, and stress management system very seriously and to constantly work at improving your on-the-job performance. This is the only way you will have the stamina, health, and clarity of mind to consistently clear the bar.

PART TWO

The Strategic Plan for Optimum Health

8

Learn the Basics about Heart Disease

The foundation of performance and longevity is good health. Yet, as a nation, we have never been so unhealthy. Obesity, cardiovascular disease, type 2 diabetes, hypertension, cancer, and many other serious diseases are rising at rates that have now reached epidemic proportions.

The reason for this rise is that most people really do not know what constitutes a healthy lifestyle. Our parents and our schoolteachers never taught us—they don't know either—and the great majority of us do not have wellness programs in our workplace. Nor do we understand how to monitor our health and our risk factors as we grow older. Somehow we have developed the misconception that staying vigorous and healthy is an intuitive process. But how can we know what is true and what is not true when there is so much confusing information about nutrition, exercise, and disease process out there in the media? Who and what are we to believe?

That is why it is so important to have the proper tools for health evaluation. During my twenty-five years of experience with thousands of clients as a performance enhancement and fitness consultant I have come to clearly understand the definitions of good health and poor health because I have seen these scenarios played out so many times over the decades. And the dozens of top medical professionals I have worked with over the years and continue to work with through my PEP (Performance Enhancement Program) and through Ochsner Clinic Foundation have helped to acquaint me intimately with the science behind state-of-the-art health care and health evaluation.

To understand the care and attention your body requires at every stage of life, it is important to know where you are at each moment of your life continuum. What is your health age versus your chronological age versus your performance age? Are you a thirty-year-old with the health of a fifty-five-year-old? Or a fifty-year-old with the body and cardiovascular system of a thirty-five-year-old? In the pages that follow, I will offer you several important criteria that will help you to evaluate accurately your health and whether you are at risk for certain disease factors. These criteria include your cardiovascular risk factors, your Body Mass Index (BMI), your waist measurement, and your body composition.

Find Your Weak Link

It is not as easy as you think to ascertain your level of fitness because the appearance of health is not always the same as true health. I remember when Frank Warren, then a thirteen-year veteran with the New Orleans Saints, dropped out of football to coach. After a while, Frank decided to get back into the game because he felt that he was better than most of the players he was coaching. When Frank came to me for preseason training, he looked as if he were in decent shape. But the in-depth health evaluation that I recommend for all of my trainees showed that he had developed coronary problems and needed angioplasty. If Frank had stepped onto the playing field without assessing his health profile, there is a strong chance that he would have died on the field.

Your career and your passion might be calling to you to put forth your most energetic effort, but no one should ever jump into the stresses of life's battles without a clear understanding of whether or not there is a weak link in your health chain—a point at which you could literally break down. Following a recent decision by the office of the commissioner of Major League Baseball to create a division known as Umpire Medical Services to manage the health of their umpires, my PEP program was hired as a consultant. I discovered that one umpire, whose weight had soared to 357 pounds, didn't know that he had type 2 diabetes.

When this man didn't want to consider the health ramifications he was facing if he didn't lose weight and begin eating and exercising right, I appealed to his better judgment. "How can you be calling the balls and the strikes for every player when you won't look at your own score? Your body already has two strikes against it. The next one could be your last." I explained how easy—and even likely—it was for him to develop complications such as heart disease that might lead to premature death. Finally he took my suggestions seriously. He lost weight and reduced his waist measurement, thereby getting his blood sugar back to normal. Amazingly, he accomplished all this without taking medication, just by following my nutrition, exercise, and lifestyle management programs.

Many people are walking time bombs and don't even know it. If you don't have the internal physical health to deal with the stresses, demands, and performance standards of your personal life and career, then it doesn't matter if you look as if you are fine or even feel relatively good.

Coronary Disease: The Number One Cause of Death

I am going to focus on coronary disease in this chapter for two main reasons: it's the number one killer and it's the most curable.

Reason 1: Heart Disease Is the Number One Killer in the United States

Nearly 60 million Americans suffer from this illness, which accounts for 41 percent of all deaths. Although most people think of it as a man's disease, coronary disease kills more than half a million women per year. It just affects them ten to fifteen years later than the average high-risk male, with risk levels gradually increasing following menopause. Even though women have their first heart attacks later than men, they are more likely to die from them. Within one year of having an attack, 25 percent of men die, but 38 percent of women die. According to the American Heart Association, if all major forms of heart and blood vessel disease were eliminated, the average life expectancy would be increased by seven years.

To understand the prevalence of this disease, and the amount of money its treatment drains from our personal and health care resources each year, let's take a look at some of the facts and statistics related to cardiovascular disease:

- By age sixty, one out of five men and one out of seventeen women develop coronary disease.
- Nearly 15 million people have a history of heart attack and/or angina (chest pain due to coronary artery disease).
- Each year, 1.5 million people have a new or recurrent heart attack and, of these, one-third—500,000—die.
- Of those whose heart attacks are fatal, 50 to 60 percent die within one hour of the onset of symptoms.
- Stroke is the leading cause of long-term disability.
- The leading cause of death in people with diabetes is heart disease. Therefore, if you have diabetes, you are at major risk for coronary disease.
- In 1966, the estimated cost of heart disease in the United States was $66 billion. By 2002, this yearly cost will be in the $80 billion to $100 billion range.
- According to a recent article in the *Wall Street Journal,* an employee's share of company medical health care expenses is expected to rise 19 percent within the next year, an average of $38 per month for workers and $134 a month for families.
- For a substantial number of people, about 300,000 per year, sudden cardiac death represents the first, last, and only manifestation of heart disease. The only way these unfortunate people could have avoided this would be to have prevented the disease from progressing in the first place.

Reason 2: Heart Disease Is the Most Curable Disease

In spite of these grim statistics, our ability to either improve or completely prevent heart disease is very great indeed. According to Dr. Carl J. Lavie, codirector of the Cardiac Rehabilitation Program and Preventive Cardiology and head of the exercise laboratory at Ochsner Clinic Foundation:

Coronary heart disease is a very modifiable and, in many cases, preventable disease. If most people followed a program of eating a healthy diet, achieving and maintaining a healthy weight, controlling their waist circumference, regularly exercising, not smoking, and drinking alcohol in moderation, I and my colleagues would have to look for another job because we wouldn't have enough business to practice.

That's how much this disease is potentially modifiable. It would become an old person's disease as opposed to such a prevalent problem in our society.

Identify Your Risk Factors

Sadly, many patients at risk are neither identified early enough nor treated as vigorously as they should be—resulting in millions of unnecessary deaths each year. For this reason, the first and most important step in taking responsibility for evaluating the state of your health should be learning if you are at risk for cardiovascular disease. To help you to understand where you stand, what your risk factors are, and whether or not you should seek further professional evaluation, let's take a look at factors that either lead directly or indirectly to heart disease and other diseases such as type 2 diabetes and some cancers. These factors include:

- Obesity
- The Body Mass Index (BMI)
- Waist circumference
- High LDL cholesterol and low HDL cholesterol
- Elevated triglycerides
- The cluster of health indicators known as Metabolic Syndrome X

Are You Overweight or Obese? Three Criteria

Weight gain has become a problem of epic proportions in our society. In 1905, only 5 percent of the population was obese, but that figure has been growing at an alarming rate. In the last decade alone obesity has risen 8 percent. As of this writing, almost 60 percent of those over the age of twenty, about 97 million people, are either overweight or obese. Of that number, 12.5 million are severely overweight, and 2 million are morbidly obese. This means that they are at great risk for serious and life-threatening health conditions such as heart disease, stroke, diabetes, and some types of cancer.

Even though being overweight or obese is considered a health risk, it is not always easy to define what those terms mean for you. Scale weight alone is not an accurate indicator. Factors such as frame size, body type, and the ratio of fat to lean muscle must also be taken into consideration.

Let's look at some of the most important tests and factors that indicate whether you are overweight or obese and define your level of risk.

1: The Ratio of Fat to Lean Muscle

I had a forty-four-year-old client who was five feet six inches and weighed 158 pounds. She knew she wanted to lose about twenty pounds, but she didn't see herself as having a severe weight problem. When she had a professional measure her fat to lean muscle ratio, however, she found out that her body fat percentage was a whopping 34.5 percent. This made her technically obese. If nothing in her lifestyle had changed as the years passed, she would most likely have continued to gain weight and increase her health risks.

Once I placed her on a good nutrition and exercise program, she lost 22 pounds of scale weight. In terms of body composition, however, she actually lost 26.7 pounds of fat and gained 5.8 pounds of lean muscle, since her body fat percentage dropped 14 points to 20.5 percent.

The following chart defines healthy and unhealthy body fat percentages for men and women.

BODY FAT PERCENTAGE

Level	Men	Women
Excellent, very lean	<11	<14
Good/lean	11–14	14–17
Average	15–17	18–22
Fair/fat	18–22	23–27
Obese	22+	27+

Three Techniques for Measuring Body Fat

There are several methods for measuring body fat. These include:

1. **Hydrostatic weighing.** This technique is the most accurate and measures a person's mass both in and out of a tank of water. This test is based on the assumption that lean tissue is denser than fat tissue. Lean tissue will sink and fat tissue will

float. This test costs between $100 and $150 and can be performed at your local health club, hospital, university, or wellness center.

2. **Skin fold measurement with a caliper.** This involves measuring subcutaneous (under-the-skin) fat with a caliper at certain points on the body. Since this test has been around for quite some time, you can get it done at YMCAs, health clubs, dieticians' offices, physical therapy centers, schools, and universities.

3. **Anthropometric measurement.** You can do this test at home. This test is based on the assumption that fat is distributed at certain sites on the body, such as the neck, wrist, and waistline. Muscle tissue is usually found at sites such as the biceps, forearm, and calf.

The following two tests, one for males and the other for females, will help you to ascertain your percentage of body fat to lean muscle. These formulas are from Phil L. Goglia's book *Turn Up the Heat: Unlock the Fat-Burning Power of Your Metabolism* and have a plus or minus error rate of 5 percent. All you need is a cloth tape measure and a calculator.

AT-HOME BODY FAT TEST FOR MALES

Step 1: Taking Measurements

1. Height in inches   _____

2. Hips in inches   _____

3. Waist in inches   _____

4. Weight in pounds _____

Step 2: Determining Your Percentage of Body Fat

1. Multiply your hips (inches) ____ × 1.4 = ____ minus 2 = ____ (A)

2. Multiply your waist (inches) ____ × 0.72 = ____ minus 4 = ____ (B)

3. Add A plus B = _____ (C)

4. Multiply your height (inches) ____ × 0.61 = ____ (D)

5. Subtract D from C, then subtract 10 more: C – D – 10 = ____ %

   Your answer will be your approximate body fat percentage, if you are a male.

AT-HOME BODY FAT TEST FOR FEMALES

Step 1: Taking Measurements

1. Height in inches _____

2. Hips in inches _____

3. Waist in inches _____

4. Weight in pounds _____

Step 2: Determining Your Percentage of Body Fat

1. Multiply your hips (inches) ____ × 1.4 = ____ minus 1 = _____ (A)

2. Multiply your waist (inches) ____ × 0.72 = ____ minus 2 = _____ (B)

3. Add A plus B = _____ (C)

4. Multiply your height (inches) _____ × 0.61 = _____ (D)

5. Subtract D from C, then subtract 10 more: C – D – 10 = _____%

   Your answer will be your approximate body fat percentage, if you are a female.

You do not necessarily have to get your body fat to lean muscle ratio tested to know that your body composition is improving. If you have been exercising and eating properly and your clothes begin to feel looser, if you find yourself taking in your belt a notch or two, or if you observe increased strength and muscularity, you will know that you are losing fat and gaining lean muscle.

2: Body Mass Index

The Body Mass Index or BMI is another important criterion in ascertaining whether you are overweight or obese. While the BMI is not an infallible standard for determining obesity and the risk of heart disease, taken together with other factors, it is a useful tool for helping to create an accurate health profile. BMI is defined as your weight in kilograms divided by your height in meters squared. To save you the trouble of converting pounds to kilograms and inches to meters, I have done the math for you. Simply look up your BMI in the table provided. Your height can be found in the left-hand column and your weight (in pounds) runs along the top of the chart. Your BMI is where both points intersect. Because people between five feet and five feet three inches have a generally lighter frame, we have included a different chart for them.

	100	110	120	130	140	150	160	170	180	190	200	210	220	230	240	250	260	270	280
5'0"	20	22	24	26	27	29	31	33	35	37	39	41	43	45	47	49	51	53	55
5'1"	19	21	23	25	27	28	30	32	34	37	39	41	43	45	47	49	51	53	55
5'2"	19	20	22	24	26	28	29	31	33	35	36	37	39	41	43	44	46	48	50

	120	130	140	150	160	170	180	190	200	210	220	230	240	250	260	270	280	290	300
5'3"	21	23	25	27	28	30	32	34	36	37	39	41	43	44	46	48	50	51	53
5'4"	21	22	24	26	28	29	31	33	34	36	38	40	41	43	45	46	48	50	52
5'5"	20	22	23	25	27	28	30	32	33	35	37	38	40	42	43	45	47	48	50
5'6"	19	21	23	24	26	27	29	31	32	34	36	37	39	40	42	44	45	47	49
5'7"	19	20	22	24	25	27	28	30	31	33	35	36	38	39	41	42	44	46	47
5'8"	18	20	21	23	24	26	27	29	30	32	34	35	37	38	40	41	43	44	46
5'9"	18	19	21	22	24	25	27	28	30	31	33	34	36	37	38	40	41	43	44
5'10"	17	19	20	22	23	24	26	27	29	30	32	33	35	36	37	39	40	42	43
5'11"	17	18	20	21	22	24	25	27	28	29	31	32	34	35	36	38	39	41	42
6'0"	16	18	19	20	22	23	24	26	27	29	30	31	33	34	35	37	38	39	41
6'1"	16	17	19	20	21	22	24	25	26	28	29	30	32	33	34	36	37	38	40
6'2"	15	17	18	19	21	22	23	24	26	27	28	30	31	32	33	35	36	37	39
6'3"	15	16	18	19	20	21	23	24	25	26	28	29	30	31	33	34	35	36	38
6'4"	15	16	17	18	20	21	22	23	24	26	27	28	29	30	32	33	34	35	37
6'5"	14	15	17	18	19	20	21	23	24	25	26	27	29	30	31	32	33	34	36
6'6"	14	15	16	17	19	20	21	22	23	24	25	27	28	29	30	31	32	34	35

Interpret Your BMI

- *If your BMI is below 20.* Unless you are an athlete with a very high lean muscle to body fat ratio, a BMI this low might mean that you are too thin and are possibly compromising your immune system.
- *If your BMI is between 20 and 22.* This range is associated with living the longest and having the lowest incidence of serious illness.
- *If your BMI is between 22 and 25.* These numbers are still within the acceptable range and are associated with good health.
- *If your BMI is between 25 and 30.* Now you are entering the zone where there are serious health risks. A BMI this high puts you at risk for developing heart disease, stroke, type 2 diabetes, and some kinds of cancers. You should definitely lower your weight through diet and exercise.

- *If your BMI is over 30.* This is the worst-case scenario where you are definitely putting yourself at risk for all of the diseases mentioned above. It is imperative that you begin to lose weight and exercise.

Having a BMI over 25 may cause your life span to decrease significantly, according to a study done in the *New England Journal of Medicine.* If your BMI is higher than 30, your life span may decrease even more sharply. Studies show that 59 percent of American men have a BMI over 25 and almost as many women. For those who have a BMI over 35, health care costs are likely to be more than twice that of individuals with a BMI between 20 and 25. Treatment of diabetes, hypertension, and cardiovascular disease count for much of this spending.

3: Waist Circumference

One of the most important and accurate indicators of obesity, the potential for cardiac disease, and other health risks is the circumference of the waist. The reason for this is because an increased measurement in the waist always indicates an increase in abdominal fat (and the ratio of body fat to lean muscle in general). Since a pound of fat is four times the volume of a pound of lean muscle tissue, it is possible for someone's scale weight and BMI to remain the same as they get older, yet for their waist to increase as lean muscle is lost and fat storage is increased through inactivity and poor nutritional habits.

Dr. J. Pervis Milnor III, one of the authors of the book *It Can Break Your Heart,* addresses the fact that a waistline higher than 35 inches in a woman and 40 inches in a man puts one at greater risk for developing not only higher cholesterol levels which leads to coronary disease, but also type 2 diabetes. According to the National Heart, Lung, and Blood Institute, a man whose waistline is 42 inches or greater is more likely to have erectile dysfunction than his leaner counterparts.

Of course, a waist measurement of 35 inches (female) or 40 inches (male) is not always an absolute indicator of health risks. You should take into consideration factors such as height, body type, and bone structure. A 35-inch waistline on a woman who is five foot eleven inches with a large frame would represent less of a health risk than the same waist circumference on a woman who is five foot four inches with a medium frame.

The Connection between Waist Circumference and Diabetes

There is a direct correlation between fat in the abdominal region of the body and diabetes. According to the American Diabetes Association, as abdominal girth increases, so do the chances of contracting type 2 diabetes. This is due to increasing insulin resistance. In fact, 88 to 97 percent of diabetes diagnosed is the direct result of obesity. New research from Kaiser Permanente found that the fatter you are, the more likely it is that you will contract type 2 diabetes before the age of forty-five. The risk of contracting this disease rises 6 percent for every five to eight pounds of extra body fat.

The number of people who have type 2 diabetes has increased 33 percent from 1990 to 1998. According to the New Orleans *Times-Picayune,* what is most alarming about this increase is that 70 percent of new cases are individuals in their thirties. The American Diabetes Association used to suggest that people get their first diabetes test at age forty-five but is now urging people to get this test earlier because undiagnosed diabetes can cause serious damage to your eyes, kidneys, nerves, and arteries long before you realize you have the disease. According to the group's new guidelines, people with any of the following risks should get tested at age thirty if they:

- Have a relative with diabetes
- Have heart disease, high blood pressure, high triglycerides, or low HDL
- Are a woman who had gestational diabetes during pregnancy or delivered a baby weighing more than nine pounds
- Are a woman with a hormonal disorder called polycystic ovarian syndrome
- Have had a previous blood sugar test that found impaired glucose tolerance, a condition that leads to diabetes.

For a detailed analysis of how abdominal fat is related to health risks, as well as nutritional and exercise programs targeted specifically for reducing fat in that area of the body, see my book *Lose Your Love Handles.*

Cardiologist Carl J. Lavie warns that even if a patient has no prior history of heart disease, if he contracts type 2 diabetes, he will have a greater chance of dying from cardiovascular disease within the next five to ten years than a patient without diabetes who has just had a heart attack.

How to Interpret Your Full Lipid Profile

Before you fill out the Cardiovascular Risk Assessment Question-naire later in this chapter, you should understand certain terms that describe your blood chemistry. When your doctor draws blood and does something called a "full lipid profile," he or she is evaluating five basic numbers:

1. **HDL, or high-density lipid protein.** HDL is the type of choles-terol that we think of as "good" or protective. If small amounts of plaque (LDL or "bad" cholesterol) have been laid down in your blood vessels, if you have enough HDL, you will be able to dissolve this plaque and use it as an energy source.
   - A good HDL level is 40 mg/dl and above for a man.
   - A good HDL level is 50 mg/dl and above for a woman.
2. **LDL, or low-density lipid protein.** This is the "bad" type of cholesterol. It collects in your blood vessels as plaque and clogs them if you have too much floating around in your bloodstream, or if you don't have sufficient HDL to dissolve it. According to the new cholesterol standards recently pub-lished by the *Journal of the American Medical Association*:
   - An LDL of less than 100 mg/dl is optimal
   - 100–129 mg/dl is near or above optimal
   - 130–159 mg/dl is borderline high
   - 160–189 mg/dl is high
   - 190 mg/dl and up is very high

   (These LDL figures are the same for both genders.)
3. **Triglyceride level.** Triglycerides are the fats that appear in the blood immediately after a meal or snack. Normally, they are stripped of their fatty acids when they pass through various types of tissue, especially adipose (beneath-the-skin) fat and skeletal muscle. When this happens, they are converted into stored energy that is gradually released and metabolized between meals according to the metabolic needs of your body. Almost everyone loves sugars and other kinds of carbo-hydrates. Unfortunately, if you are insulin sensitive and eat more carbohydrates than you require daily, your triglyceride level will elevate. When this happens, your disease risk for hypoglycemia and type 2 diabetes can increase and you will become more susceptible to coronary disease.

- A normal triglyceride level is 150 or below.
- 150–199 is borderline high.
- 200–499 is high.
- 500 or over is very high.
4. **Total cholesterol.** This number is found by adding your HDL plus your LDL plus your triglycerides, then dividing that sum by five. Ideally, your total cholesterol should be 100 plus your age.
   - A total cholesterol less than 200 mg/dl is desirable
   - 200–239 mg/dl is borderline high
   - 240 mg/dl or higher is considered high
5. **Ratio between your total cholesterol and your HDL.**
   - The average male has a 3.5–1 ratio
   - The average female has a 4.5–1 ratio
   - The average athlete has a 2.1–1 to a 2.8–1 ratio

Assessing Cardiac Risk Factors

Now that you understand the basic vocabulary and health indicators, you are ready to take the Cardiovascular Risk Assessment Questionnaire and the Metabolic Syndrome X Questionnaire. If after filling out these questionnaires you find yourself in a moderate- to high-risk group, I urge you to go to your doctor for a professional evaluation and immediate care. Heart disease is too serious to ignore.

Cardiovascular Risk Assessment Questionnaire

To determine your major cardiovascular risk factors, add the number of positive risk factors and subtract the number of negative risk factors to get a total.

- If you have only *one* of these risk factors, your risk of major cardiovascular disease within the next ten years is *slightly* increased (approximately 5 percent).
- If you have *two* major risk factors, your risk is *moderately* increased (approximately 10 percent).
- If you have *three* major risk factors, your risk of major cardiovascular disease within the next ten years is *markedly* increased (approximately 20 percent or higher).

Positive Risk Factors

	Yes	No
1. Do you have a family history of major cardio-vascular disease in first-degree relatives (parents and grandparents) who are younger than fifty-five years old if you are male or younger than sixty-five years old if you are female?	☐	☐
2. Are you currently smoking, have you smoked within the last three years, or do you smoke more than twenty packs a year?	☐	☐
3. Hypertension—Is your blood pressure greater than 140/90 mmHg or are you taking antihypertensive medication?	☐	☐
4. Obesity—Is your BMI greater than 25? (See table for calculating BMI on page 89.)	☐	☐
5. Obesity—Is your waist circumference greater than 40 inches if you are male, or 35 inches if you are female? (See page 90.)	☐	☐
6. Do you have high LDL (bad) cholesterol—greater than 160 mg/dl?	☐	☐
7. Do you have low HDL cholesterol—less than 40 mg/dl in men and less than 50 mg/dl in women?	☐	☐
8. Do you have elevated triglycerides greater than 200 mg/dl?	☐	☐
9. Are you physically inactive, that is, do you exercise less than thirty minutes one time per week?	☐	☐

Total yes answers _____

Negative Risk Factors

	Yes	No
1. Is your HDL (good) cholesterol greater than 60 mg/dl?	☐	☐
2. Do you exercise for thirty minutes at a time at least four times per week?	☐	☐

Total yes answers _____

Metabolic Syndrome X Questionnaire

There are five main measurements that are listed as risk factors for Metabolic Syndrome X. If you have three of the five following metabolic syndrome risk factors, your risk of major cardiovascular disease during the next ten years is at least moderately increased. Please check off the ones that apply.

	Yes	No
1. Do you have a waist circumference greater than forty inches if you are a man or greater than thirty-five inches if you are a woman?	☐	☐
2. Do you have hypertension that is being medically treated or blood pressure greater than 135/85 mm/Hg?	☐	☐
3. Are your triglycerides greater than 150 mg/dl?	☐	☐
4. Do you have a low HDL value, that is, less than 40 mg/dl if you are a man or less than 50 mg/dl if you are a woman?	☐	☐
5. Do you have a fasting glucose greater than 110 mg/dl?	☐	☐

If you have diabetes mellitus that is under treatment or a fasting blood sugar greater than 126 mg/dl, your risk of major cardiovascular disease during the next ten years is markedly increased, in excess of 20 percent. In fact, a patient with diabetes who has no prior history of heart disease has a greater chance of dying from cardiovascular disease during the next five to ten years than a patient without diabetes who has just had a heart attack. The risk of major events related to heart disease is increased even further if the patient with diabetes has two or more of the other major risk factors.

All of these factors are considered general and should be a part of every standard risk assessment for adult patients. Tests for all of these factors are covered by all insurance companies or health maintenance organizations.

Further Define Your Overall Cardiac Risk

There are additional tests you can request from your doctor that can further define your overall cardiovascular risk. But since some of these are not covered by health insurance plans, keep in mind that you will likely have to pay for some of them yourself. These tests are discussed in detail on Dr. Carl J. Lavie's Web site www.myheartrisk.com, which also provides a test that automatically calculates your risk of heart disease.

The hs-CRP test. One of the newer risk factors to be discovered is hs-CRP, which stands for high-sensitivity C-reactive protein. Hs-CRP is measured by a blood test and is a very accurate maker for small levels of inflammation in the body. Low levels of inflammation often accompany atherosclerosis and are usually present to a greater degree in individuals likely to develop future heart attacks and strokes. In studies of healthy men and women, as well as those who already have heart disease, hs-CRP has been shown to be at least as useful, if not more useful, than cholesterol levels in predicting future heart attack and stroke. When you combine measurements of cholesterol levels with your hs-CRP score and your other risk factors, the ability to predict your risk of future heart attack increases markedly.

The low cost of this test, about $20 to $50 in most labs, makes it a fairly common tool for additional risk assessment. It should be covered by most health plans.

Lipoprotein(a) test. Lipoprotein(a) is a particle that is structurally very similar to LDL, or bad cholesterol. Although your Lp(a) values are influenced by your genetics, levels are generally higher in the elderly, in African-Americans, and in women. Elevated levels of Lp(a) may increase vascular disease risk by inhibiting the body's ability to dissolve clots, by playing a role in "foam cell" formation—an early step in the atherosclerosis process—and in increasing oxidative stress. Oxidative stress is often referred to as the body's rust and can be seen in the little brown "age marks" that you have on the back of your hands.

Although most studies have shown that an elevated Lp(a) alone is a risk factor for cardiovascular disease, your risk will be particularly increased when you also have elevated total cholesterol or LDL levels.

While Lp(a) is not considered a standard lab test, it should be covered by most standard health plans. Dr. Carl J. Lavie recommends it to the following types of patients:

- Those who have symptoms of vascular disease without other risk factors.

- Those who have symptoms of vascular disease out of proportion to their risk factor profiles.
- Patients who are borderline for drug treatment for lipids (cholesterol), meaning those who do not have a very good profile, but are not quite bad enough to meet current guidelines for drug treatment.
- Patients who have not only a mildly increased LDL value but also have a mildly increased triglyceride level and a mildly reduced HDL value.
- Patients whose cholesterol shows only minimal improvement when taking statin medications. Sometimes these individuals are found to have very high Lp(a) values, greater than 100 mg/dl.

Homocysteine test. Elevated levels of homocysteine may increase the risk of vascular disease. Elevated levels of homocysteine have been associated with increased risk of venous thrombosis, pulmonary embolism, peripheral vascular disease, cerebral vascular disease, and coronary artery disease.

Although homocysteine levels may be determined by genetic factors, higher levels are associated with decreased fitness; a low intake of vitamins B6 and B12, which contain folic acid; and renal failure.

A homocysteine test can cost as little as $50 or as much as $125.

Stress testing. According to the American Heart Association and the American College of Cardiology (ACC), there are no absolute guidelines to doing a stress test in a patient unless he or she is showing symptoms of chest pain or shortness of breath. Therefore, many health plans may not pay for this unless symptoms appear. However, many physicians recognize that a "positive" or abnormal stress test can indicate a significant increase in risk when combined with several other risk factors. This can range from four to eighty times an increase in risk.

For this reason, many clinicians interested in preventive medicine feel that a stress test is reasonable for:

- Men older than forty, and particularly men above fifty years of age, especially with two or more risk factors
- Postmenopausal women who have two major risk factors

- Sedentary middle-aged individuals who are about to start an exercise program more vigorous than regular walking

If your insurance does not cover this kind of test, it will cost you $450 for a simple echocardiogram (ECG), $800 for a cardiopulmonary test, $1,000 for an exercise echo, and $2,700 for a nuclear stress test.

Coronary calcium scanning. Substantial research data indicate that an electron beam CT scanning for coronary calcium deposits can be of great use in identifying early atheriosclerosis and potential risk factors for CAD (coronary artery disease). Since the cost of this test is high (between $400 and $800) and the American Heart Association does not recommend its routine use, most insurance companies do not pay for this test at the present time. However, if you decide to have a coronary calcium scan performed, be aware that a value in the 10 to 100 range is considered high and should be followed by more vigorous risk factor modification and possibly treadmill testing (especially for values greater than 100–200).

Should You Consider These Tests?

In general, cardiologist Carl J. Lavie recommends that any individual who has two or more major risk factors, can afford the costs, and is interested in reducing his or her major cardiovascular risk, might at least consider getting the hs-CRP, Lp(a), and homocysteine tests, in addition to other standard testing for cardiovascular disease.

Recently, a client named Susan signed up for my PEP program. When we administered the standard health and screening portion of my program, we discovered that she had a total cholesterol slightly less than 200 and a borderline high LDL of 130. In the past, most doctors would have just given her some dietary recommendations or possibly put her on statin medications and then not worried about her. However, when Dr. Lavie discovered that Susan had some history of early death from heart disease in her family, he recommended that she be tested for these other three blood factors. When the results came back, we discovered that Susan had elevated levels of Lp(a), a hereditary factor that put her at greater risk for developing vascular disease. When Susan was given an angiogram after several other tests including stress testing were abnormal, sure enough,

Dr. Lavie found blockages in her arteries. In other words, this test quite possibly saved her life.

Take Ownership of Your Health

One question I ask all my clients is: "Do you live as if you rent your body or as if you own it?" Far too many of us treat our bodies as if they were rental apartments. And when you are merely renting a living space, you will never take as much responsibility for its upkeep as you would with a home you owned. If you want to achieve optimum health, it is time to start taking ownership of your body, and not treating it as a transient space that you rent.

9

Two Essential Strategies to Cut Your Risk of Heart Disease

Now that you have an idea about your risk factors, be reassured that there are certain specific actions you can take to greatly reduce or prevent your risk of cardiovascular disease. The three most important are exercise, dietary modification, and learning how to manage stress. As usual, always consult with your doctor before undertaking any exercise or nutritional modifications in your lifestyle.

Strategy 1: Exercise for Heart Health

Although I discuss the benefits of exercise fully in chapter 11, be aware that doing the right kind of exercise is one of the best prescriptions for gaining and maintaining a healthy heart and cardiovascular system. I will just hit the high points in this chapter.

According to an excellent ten-year study done at the Ochsner Heart and Vascular Institute:

- Regular exercise is associated with marked reductions in the long-term risks for major cardiac events such as heart attack or stroke, and death from heart disease.
- People who exercise regularly, at least three times per week, reduced their chance of a cardiac event from 30 to 50 percent.

- A study from the Cooper Clinic shows that physical fitness is directly correlated with increased life span and fewer deaths from cardiovascular causes and cancer.
- Even for obese individuals or for people with several coronary heart disease risk factors, physical fitness strongly decreases the chance of developing symptoms of heart disease.

The Ochsner Heart and Vascular Institute has found that the following types of exercise are most effective in treating people with cardiovascular disease, or for people wishing to avoid developing cardiovascular disease:

- Dynamic or aerobic exercises, which include walking, running, cycling, swimming, aerobic dancing, cross-country skiing, and using elliptical machines.
- Light isotonic exercises such as using handgrips or weight lifting (frequent repetitions with low amounts of weight).

The Pro Circuit Exercise Program, which I describe in chapter 13, fills this prescription perfectly in that it alternates periods of aerobic exercise with periods of isotonic (weight training) exercise.

But before beginning any exercise program, if you are a healthy but sedentary woman over the age of fifty or a man over the age of forty, remember that the American College of Sports Medicine recommends that you should always consult with your physician and have a preexercise medical examination. This is even more important if you have high blood pressure, chest pains, high cholesterol, or any serious risk factors for heart disease, or if you are a smoker.

Strategy 2: Eat Right and Take the Proper Supplements for Heart Health

In general, the best food program for cardiovascular health is what is loosely referred to as the Mediterranean diet—lots of fresh fruits, vegetables, lean meats, and cold-water fish such as salmon, trout, or mackeral that are rich in omega-3 and omega-6 fatty acids. I have included in chapter 10 an extensive food program for readers to adapt to their needs. Here, however, I'd like to list some of the recommendations that Ochsner cardiologist Dr. Carl J. Lavie uses with his patients, since these are specific for improving or maintaining cardiovascular health.

1. *Consume alcohol in moderate amounts.* Excess alcohol has deleterious effects upon the health, including alcoholism, cirrhosis of the liver, various cancers (particularly breast cancer and colon cancer), hypertension, stroke, family stress, and accidental death from causes such as automobile accidents. However, a recent analysis of fifty-one major studies has shown that individuals who drink up to 20 grams of alcohol (one or two drinks) per day had a 20 percent lower risk of major coronary events when compared to those who abstained from drinking. Other studies have shown that moderate alcohol consumption can lower the risk of heart disease from 25 to 40 percent. Other benefits include the lowering of risk for diseases such as strokes from blood clots, hardening of the arteries in the limbs, congestive heart failure, and type 2 diabetes.

   While the mechanism behind alcohol's protective role is still somewhat unclear, it seems to be related to increasing HDL levels (good cholesterol), preventing blood clotting, and having beneficial effects on insulin activity. Studies have shown that having a low HDL level is one of the most important risk factors in heart disease.

   Wine, particularly red wine, is more effective in reducing heart disease than beer or other types of alcoholic beverages. The reason for this is that red wine contains a number of chemicals that have antioxidant effects.

2. *Eat lots of fiber.* Many studies have shown that dietary fiber, particularly soluble fiber, has a number of beneficial effects on the cardiovascular system. Fiber also reduces the risk of colon and breast cancer. Dietary fiber reduces not only levels of cholesterol but it also reduces:
   - High insulin levels
   - High glucose values
   - Hypertension
   - Obesity
   - Various clotting parameters.

   (See chapter 10 for ways to include fiber in your daily diet and for suggestions on the best types of fiber to eat.)

3. *Lower cholesterol and increase immunity with soy.* The American Heart Association recommends that people eat 20 grams of soy protein per day to lower their cholesterol levels. Soy is also

helpful in the production of hormones and can stimulate estrogen production in menopausal women. Other studies indicate that soy may actually help the immune system and protect against cancer. Societies such as Japan that ingest large amounts of soy protein in their diets have significantly lower levels of cancer than we do in the United States.

Soy is found in tofu and cheeses made with soy protein. I recommend to many clients soy protein powder, which can be made into a delicious shake by adding milk or juice.

4. *Reduce your risk with omega-3 fatty acids.* Many studies have shown that patients with cardiovascular disease who ingest omega-3 fatty acids (EPA and DHA fish oils), either taken as supplements or in cold-water fish such as salmon or mackeral, have seen a marked reduction in their risk for cardiovascular disease. According to Dr. Carl J. Lavie, studies published in recent years have shown that heart patients who take omega-3 fatty acids show some improvement in cholesterol levels and a 20 to 70 percent reduction in death rates. Dr. Lavie prescribes 1,000 mg combined of both EPA and DHA for his heart patients.

5. *Strengthen your heart health with antioxidants.* The oxidation of LDL cholesterol by free radicals plays a major role in the formation, progression, and rupture of plaques involved in heart attacks and stroke. Antioxidants include vitamin E (400 to 800 IU/day), vitamin C (500 to 1,000 mg/day), selenium, coenzyme Q10, lycopene, and falconoid. Several studies have shown that antioxidants have the potential to interfere in each step of these processes by inhibiting oxidant formation in the first place, by interfering in the oxidant activity that has already taken place, and even by helping to repair areas of oxidation-induced injuries to the walls of the arteries.

However, the jury is still out on whether antioxidants are as strong a force to prevent heart disease as the media generally purports. Studies have shown that people who take antioxidants also consume large amounts of fruits, vegetables, and dietary fiber; eat lower amounts of saturated fats; are often more physically active; and have healthier living habits. However, as Dr. Carl J. Lavie says, there is no harm in taking antioxidants and possibly some positive benefits, particularly for patients with high levels of oxidative stress. But antioxidants should be considered only one dietary factor in the treatment and prevention of heart disease.

6. *Reduce your homocysteine level.* The evidence supporting the importance of the relationship between levels of homocysteine, an amino acid that circulates in the blood, and the risk of cardiovascular disease has been increasing in recent years. Homocycsteine is affected by three important B vitamins: folic acid, B6, and B12. Numerous studies have shown that patients with heart disease have higher levels of homocysteine and lower levels of B6 and B12 than healthy people. The risk of vascular disease significantly increases when levels are in the 12 to 13 micromoles/liter, and especially when levels reach higher than 15.

The best way to lower levels of homocysteine is to supplement your daily diet with folic acid. The typical person in the United States ingests an average of 50 to 100 micrograms of folic acid per day, just in the foods he or she eats. Dr. Carl J. Lavie suggests supplementing that with an extra 400 mg, which can be accomplished by taking a commercial multivitamin such as Centrum, Theragram, or one recommended by your local health foods store. Although B6 and B12 are available in small amounts in most commercial multivitamins, Dr. Lavie highly recommends taking Folgard from Upsher-Smith. This vitamin contains not only a significant amount of B6 and B12 (greater than other multivitamins), but also contains 800 mg of folic acid. Or you may wish to ask your doctor to prescribe a multivitamin for you, since pharmaceutical-quality supplements are superior to over-the-counter medications.

Exercise also decreases the levels of homocysteine in the blood.

Turn Your Life Around

Every day in my Performance Enhancement Program at Elmwood Fitness Center, I am inspired by the number of people who prove that making intelligent lifestyle changes can make a significant difference in their overall health and quality of life.

Forty-five-year-old Ray has a high-profile, high-pressure position with a local telecommunications company. When he first came to me he was overweight, suffered from the effects of stress, had borderline high blood pressure, and had gout. He was also experiencing chronic exhaustion. "By the end of the day when I got home, I would be totally wiped out," Ray lamented. He knew it was time to make a lifestyle change if he wanted to reclaim his health, reduce his risk of cardiovascular disease, and improve his quality of life and performance levels.

Ray joined my program at the Elmwood Fitness Center and started with a full health evaluation. Then we placed him with a personal trainer and made an appointment for him to meet with a nutritionist to set up a food program. "Within the second month of the program," Ray said, "I really started to see results, and by the third month, the changes were really dramatic." Ray, who is six feet two inches, went from 225 pounds with a body fat percentage of 26 to a lean 200 pounds with a body fat percentage of 12. He got off the gout medication, dropped his blood pressure to within acceptable levels, lowered his cholesterol and triglycerides, and began to experience a tremendous increase in energy.

While Ray sometimes cheats a little on the nutritional program, he always goes back to eating right because of the way it makes him feel—great. And he's religious about doing his weekly workouts. At this point he's even doing more than I recommend, up to an hour and a half, four days a week. "I'm in the best shape I've been in since high school," he enthused. "Some of my friends have been walking up to me, grabbing my arm, and saying, 'Man, what are you doing?' They can see that I've bulked up pretty good. It's a great program and it's just so easy to get into the flow of the work. And before you know it, you're seeing results." Recently Ray entered the race for mayor of his hometown and won. This man is a winner on all fronts.

10

The Nutritional Program
for the Twenty-first Century

Regain Your Focus through Proper Nutrition

New Orleans boasts one of the finest cuisines in the world. Unfortunately, the high fat content of these savory dishes can be very hard on one's health. I once had a client named Kirk who ran political campaigns, which, as you can well imagine, involves a great deal of wheeling and dealing at fund-raising banquets and a good deal of entertaining in top restaurants. It also involves a high degree of stress, since politics in New Orleans is unusually cutthroat.

When Kirk came to me he was already obese, with a waist measurement and body fat percentage well over the norm. Since I worked with many athletes and clients who are constantly on the road, I had become an expert at how to eat nutritiously in restaurants. I coached Kirk in the nutritional principles outlined in this chapter, teaching him how to use food to keep his energy levels consistent. When his blood sugar levels stayed at a healthy and steady level, he dealt better with stress because his brain, which is the biggest user of glucose in the body, always had a steady supply. He was able to stay focused and make quick decisions in what we in New Orleans call "political war." By eating a healthier food plan, he lost seventy-five pounds and decreased his body fat percentage, thereby lowering his disease risk factors.

Today Kirk is a happier, calmer, and healthier man through proper nutrition. And he intends to stay that way.

The first step in my program for greater health and performance is proper nutrition. Whether you need to lose weight, gain weight and greater muscle mass because you are underweight, or seriously change your nutritional lifestyle to reduce your risk of diseases such as heart attack, high cholesterol, hypertension, or type 2 diabetes, this chapter will provide you with a food program that will meet your nutritional needs. Once you begin following a food plan that shows you how to eat the appropriate number of calories for your performance and nutritional needs, and the proper *types* of food from the three main food groups, you will begin to see marked results in as few as thirty days. Your scale weight will drop an average of two pounds per week, your body fat will decrease, you will see a thinner waistline and more lean muscle. For optimum results in health, stamina, and strength, you should follow any food and exercise program for a minimum of twelve weeks.

Keep in mind, however, that this is not a fad *diet*, which, by definition, is a calorically deprived food regimen that no one could remain on for very long without significant health ramifications, stress, and hunger. This is a food program you can follow for a *lifetime*. Coupled with my stress reduction and exercise programs, this nutritional program for the twenty-first century is designed not only to help you achieve your ideal weight and body composition goals, but also to dramatically increase your health, performance, energy levels, and longevity. The thousands of elite athletes and ordinary men and women with whom I have worked for more than twenty-five years are living proof of this program's effectiveness.

The State of Nutritional Health in America

One has only to examine the terrible health ramifications that result from the large number of Americans who are overweight to see that most people do not understand the basics of proper nutrition. At present, 59.4 percent of adults over the age of 20—approximately 97 million people—are overweight or obese.

Contrast this figure to the one from 1900, when only 5 percent of the population was obese. Back then, people ate a healthier diet comprised of whole foods. There were no supermarkets filled with low-calorie, low-fat, or processed foods. Fad diets had barely been invented, and significantly fewer people had jobs that forced them to be physically inactive.

These days 40 percent of all women and 25 percent of all men are dieting, and about one out of three people are trying to maintain their weight. According to the American College of Sports Medicine, most of these programs fail in the long run. Most people who diet do lose pounds, but on average the majority gain back 67 percent of their lost weight within a year and the remainder within five years. These individuals spend approximately $30 billion per year on commercial weight loss programs and about $6 billion on weight loss products.

Medical treatments and workdays lost because of obesity-related illnesses cost us over $100 billion per year. Even if you are a person who takes good care of yourself through proper nutrition and exercise, you will still end up absorbing these expenses due to rising insurance costs in your company health plans.

There is hope, however, that we can turn this trend around. Even though more than 250,000 deaths a year are caused by obesity-related health problems, obesity is the *second greatest preventable cause of death* in the United States. (As stated in chapter 8, heart disease is the first.) As we have seen, many major risk factors for disease are directly related to weight issues, such as waistline circumference, high cholesterol, BMI, and body fat percentage.

The Seven Myths about Weight Loss

The first step toward good nutrition is to separate the myths and misconceptions about food, weight loss, and health from the simple facts of proper food programming. Much of the information we read and watch in the media is not founded on truth or on sound scientific thinking. Let's begin by looking at some of our culture's widely held notions about metabolism, weight loss, and caloric needs.

Myth 1: You can only lose weight if you eat fewer calories. The less you eat, the more you lose. While it is true that eating fewer calories than your metabolism requires will initially help you to lose weight, any low-calorie diet will eventually result in diminishing returns. The reason for this is evolutionary. For most of their history human beings have been hunter-gatherers whose food supply was directly proportional

to their success at hunting or foraging. During times of food short-
ages, the human body learned to slow down its metabolism and store
fat as a protective hedge against starvation. According to Dr. Ann de
Wees Allen of the Glycemic Research Institute, whenever a woman
eats fewer than 1,200 calories a day or a man fewer than 1,650, fat-
storing enzymes in the body are automatically triggered.

If you eat a low-calorie diet for any extended time, several
unpleasant side effects will result. First, as the body strives to adjust
its needs to what it perceives as famine, weight loss will stop. Eventually, your starved body will start feeding off its own muscle tissue to
receive essential nutrients, creating an increasing ratio of fat to lean
muscle. If you try to exercise while on a very low-calorie diet, you will
not have the nutritional support necessary to repair and build muscle tissue. A low caloric intake will also cause fatigue and irritability.

Myth 2: Scale weight is an accurate indication of how thin you are. Many
people think that simply having a low scale weight automatically
ensures that they are healthy. But a low scale weight is not an accurate indicator of whether or not you have a healthy body composition. It is possible to weigh the "right" amount for your height and
body type yet still have an unhealthy amount of body fat. My nutritionist, Molly Kimball, calls those types of individuals "skinny fat
people." Many vegetarians, who eat relatively little protein, are thin
but have a high body fat content. One woman who is five feet eight
inches weighed only 158 pounds, but she had a body fat percentage
of 34.25, which made her technically obese and at risk for significant
health deterioration as she got older.

Many people do not gain weight as they age, but they lose lean
tissue and begin to collect fat in the abdominal area. One seven-year
study cited in the *Canadian Journal of Diabetes Care* showed that even
though the subjects' scale weight and BMI remained the same as
they got older, there was a significant increase in their waist measurements, accompanied by a 30 percent increase in abdominal fat. This
greater waistline and body fat percentage made them prime candi-
dates for diseases such as type 2 diabetes.

On the other hand, I know of people who are overweight but
carry a significant amount of muscle tissue in relation to their body
fat. They have low cholesterol, good triglyceride levels, and high
energy and performance levels because they exercise regularly and
have learned how to eat nutritionally. While it would be optimal for

them to lose some of that weight, overall they are actually healthier and have a higher level of cardiovascular fitness than the skinny person who has low muscle mass and high body fat content.

How much metabolically active tissue—lean muscle—you have is more indicative of your health profile than the mere appearance of thinness.

Myth 3: You can still lose weight if you don't exercise. Many diet books downplay the importance of exercise, claiming that all you need to do to lose weight is to eat a nutritional, low-calorie food plan. Studies have shown, however, that unless you make exercise a part of your lifestyle, it is likely that you will gain back all your lost weight within six months of going off the diet.

The American College of Sports Medicine says that making exercise and cardiovascular training a part of your lifestyle significantly increases your metabolism, helping you to lose unwanted weight faster and to build more lean muscle tissue. According to several of the studies they have published, it is the only way to keep off lost weight over the long term.

Myth 4: Eating carbohydrates will make you gain weight. Many popular diet plans warn people to stay away from carbohydrates because they are "fattening." Whether or not a food is a carbohydrate is irrelevant. Everyone needs a certain percentage of fats, proteins, and carbohydrates in their daily diet. What matters is what kind of carbohydrate you choose, simple or complex, which determines how quickly or slowly a carb digests and how long it takes to release its food energy in the body. Simple carbohydrates such as sugary desserts digest quickly. Therefore a higher percentage of these types of food will be stored as fat, since the body cannot use them so fast. On the other hand, complex carbohydrates such as sweet potatoes, bran muffins, brown rice, yams, and multigrain bread digest very slowly and therefore can be more fully utilized as an energy source.

Myth 5: Fats make you fat, so avoid them. Everyone needs a certain percentage of fats in their daily food program to keep them healthy and nutritionally balanced. In fact, fats are an excellent energy source. Not all fats are created equal, however. For example, you should choose monounsaturated fats such as olive oil above saturated fats (see page 117 for a thorough discussion of fats).

Most people do not realize that the low-fat foods they buy in the supermarket are not "health foods." They are actually filled with hidden sugars such as honey, molasses, maltodextrin, and fructose. Otherwise, they would have no flavor. So don't avoid fats. Just learn to eat the proper amounts and types.

Myth 6: Some people are simply doomed to be overweight because of genetics. Many people believe that they are overweight because they have inherited the dreaded "fat gene." Often these individuals can even point to their overweight families as proof of the hopelessness of their condition. While there are those rare individuals who are heavy because of genetic factors, such as someone with a family history of thyroid problems, most of the time one's genetic heritage does not give the whole picture.

In my experience, environmental factors such as lifestyle, quantities and types of foods ingested (too much or too little), how much sleep you get each night, your stress level, how frequently you eat, and how much you exercise should always be evaluated if you have a chronic weight problem. I almost always find that people who believe they simply cannot lose weight do not have a clear understanding that real and permanent weight loss is a lifestyle issue made up of many factors working in tandem.

Myth 7: Low-calorie foods are good for you. Many people believe that low-calorie food products are generally more healthy than ordinary foods—and supermarket shelves are filled with processed foods labeled "low-cal." The danger, however, is that low-calorie often means "empty calories"—a lot of food volume with limited nutritional value. Eating these types of foods may fill you up temporarily, but they will not adequately support your body's nutritional needs. In fact, eating too many low-calorie foods usually triggers a higher level of food cravings as your body tries to signal its need for more nutritionally satisfying foods.

Calories are not the enemy. They are simply heat-energy units that the body uses either as an energy source or to repair tissue. Each person has a particular daily caloric requirement, based on what he or she needs for bodily repair, daily activity, and exercise. If you do not ingest enough calories to adequately fuel and support your metabolic functions, your body will eventually begin to cannibalize its own muscle tissue to get the nutrients it so desperately needs.

Now that we have separated the facts about nutrition from some of the most common myths, let's take an in-depth look at the basic components behind a well-designed food program.

Food Programming versus Dieting

I am often amazed at how little understanding people have of the roles played by all three food groups—carbohydrates, proteins, and fats—in the maintenance of physical health. Popular diet books only add to this confusion. Some diet authors advocate an almost total avoidance of carbohydrates and a large intake of protein. Some give readers the idea that all fats are bad. Others downplay the importance of choosing unsaturated fats such as olive oil and soy butter, over saturated fats such as dairy butter and cheese, by including recipes with heavy, creamy sauces in their food plans. You could probably lose weight on any of these diets, since most people eat so inconsistently that almost *any* routine food program will have a positive effect on the body's metabolic processes. But no one can stay on an extreme or unbalanced food program for long and expect to remain healthy.

The key to maintaining weight loss, eliminating health risks, increasing energy levels, maintaining performance, improving your moods, and increasing your longevity is to follow a food program that can become a lifestyle. This type of food program must have several basic characteristics:

- It must be intelligently balanced among carbohydrates, proteins, and fats, based on the evidence presented by nutritional science.
- It must adequately satisfy your body's daily caloric requirements.
- If you need to lose weight initially, it should never put your daily caloric intake so low that you will feel undue hunger, physical or emotional stress, or loss of energy.
- It should provide you with three balanced meals and at least two snacks per day to keep your energy levels consistent.
- It should have a certain amount of flexibility built into it to allow for your individual nutritional needs, since we are all a bit different from one another. For example, a man or woman who is very athletic will require more protein than your average person.

Generally, I have found that the percentages that work best for most people are 55 percent low-glycemic carbohydrates, 20 percent lean protein, and 25 percent acceptable fat. Allowing for individual differences, Dr. E. C. Henley, Ph.D., R.D., executive vice president and director of nutritional sciences for Physicians Pharmaceuticals, the experienced nutrition researcher and counselor who has designed the food program in this chapter, has built a bit of flexibility into that range. I guarantee that every reader who follows this food program will experience, in as few as thirty days, significant fat loss, an increase in lean muscle, lowered cholesterol, decreased health risks, and a marked increase in energy levels. But I also encourage you to listen to your body and observe its performance levels. For example, you might find that as you increase your level of exercise, you may need a somewhat higher percentage of lean protein. Or you may discover that you are an individual who is at his or her most energetic when you stick with 55 percent acceptable carbohydrates—or maybe even a bit more.

Let's take a look at the three food groups and the role each nutrient plays in the body.

Carbohydrates

In my experience, many people find a food program consisting of 55 percent carbohydrates an intimidating amount. This is because many of the popular diet books out there have caused people to shift their dietary fears from fats to carbohydrates. The key is not to be afraid to eat carbohydrates, but to learn how to *manage* your intake of carbs relative to your activity level. We all know of people who have lost a great deal of scale weight on low-carbohydrate diets, but it's a sure thing that they felt irritable, headachy, and fatigued while on that diet. To maintain the brain and central nervous system, the body needs a certain amount of glucose, which it gets from sugars and starches, the by-products of carbohydrates after digestion. The body stores this glucose in the liver and in the muscles. When you do not ingest a sufficient amount of carbohydrates in your daily diet, the body has to get its supply from somewhere. At that point, the body will begin breaking down its own muscle protein to synthesize glucose to provide your vital organs with an adequate supply. The weight you will lose on a low-carbohydrate diet will be muscle tissue, not fat, because your body cannot break down its fat stores into glucose.

The goal of any good weight loss program should always be to lose as little muscle as possible in comparison to fat loss. For every gram of muscle tissue you lose, you lose 4 grams of water. For every gram of fat lost, you lose only 1 gram of water. Water weight is not true long-term weight loss, because water is the easiest thing in the world to gain back. If, after losing weight on a diet, you start eating a larger amount of carbohydrates during times of stress, the body will quickly regain its lost muscle tissue and its associated water weight.

Remember, the goal of any nutrition program should be to spare lean muscle tissue at the expense of excess body fat. Keep in mind also that a pound of fat is four times the volume of a pound of lean muscle, so losing pounds of fat will create the greatest transformation in your physical appearance. So don't be afraid of carbohydrates. This does not mean, however, that you can eat all the carbohydrates you want. A recent study at Stanford University School of Medicine showed that eating a diet extremely high in carbohydrates caused triglycerides (bad fats) to go up. It is possible to have too much of a good thing. The key is balance.

Remember, all carbohydrates are not created equal. Complex carbohydrates such as sweet potatoes, yams, brown rice, and whole grains will be utilized more efficiently by the body than simple sugars such as candy and cakes. I'm not saying that you can never again indulge your sweet tooth, but it is important to eat desserts in moderation. Make them a special treat, not a daily occurrence.

Another factor to consider when choosing appropriate carbohydrates is their rating on the Glycemic Index. Foods with a high glycemic rating stimulate a higher than normal production of insulin in the body and tend to stimulate fat storage. Foods that have a low glycemic rating do not significantly elevate insulin or stimulate fat storage. High glycemic foods should be avoided or eaten in moderation.

The following are the twenty carbohydrate foods most frequently eaten by Americans and their Glycemic Index, followed by a list of acceptable glycemic foods. These lists were provided by the Glycemic Research Institute.

Top Twenty Carbohydrates Ingested by Americans	*Glycemic Index*
1. Potatoes	High
2. White bread	High
3. Cold breakfast cereal	High

Top Twenty Carbohydrates

Ingested by Americans	*Glycemic Index*
4. Dark bread	High
5. Orange juice	High but acceptable in ½ cup serving
6. Banana	High
7. White rice	High
8. Pizza	Very high
9. Pasta	Acceptable
10. Muffins	High
11. Fruit punch	High
12. Coca-Cola (regular)	High
13. Apple	Acceptable
14. Skim milk	Acceptable
15. Pancakes	High
16. Table sugar (sucrose)	High
17. Jam (containing sugar)	High
18. Cranberry juice (containing sugar)	High
19. French fries	High
20. Candy	High

Acceptable (Low) Glycemic Foods

Apple	Reduced-fat ice cream
Applesauce (unsweetened)	Spaghetti and meatballs
Blueberries	Hot and sour soup/Egg drop soup
Blackberries	Chicken lo mein
Cherries	Pound cake (one slice)
Orange	Sweet potatoes
Peach	Swiss Miss hot cocoa, no sugar added
Pear	Diet VeryFine Ice Tea Mix
Libby's Natural Lite Pear Halves	Newman's Own All Natural Salsa
Avocado salad	Shrimp cocktail with sauce
McDonald's scrambled eggs	Curried chicken salad
Smucker's Natural Creamy Peanut Butter	Sponge cake (two slices)
	Ravioli, meat filled
Stouffer's Lean Cuisine Chicken Primavera	Hellmann's Creamy Caesar Dressing

For a more extensive list of high and low glycemic index foods, please see my book *Lose Your Love Handles.*

Proteins

I suggest a daily intake of 20 percent lean protein. Good sources of protein are chicken breasts, all types of fish, beef with a low fat content (in moderation), and soy products. Protein is a stabilizing food that assists in insulin management, as well as serves other vital roles in normal body function. Because protein is not stored, a person requires three balanced meals and two or three snacks that include protein per day to suppress their hunger and mobilize their body fat for burning during physical exercise. A good protein to ingest as a snack would be soy-based foods such as Personal Edge soy protein powder, which you can find in many health food stores or General Nutrition Center stores in your area. Research has shown the greatest benefits occur from ingesting at least 20 to 25 grams per day. I suggest adding your soy powder to low-fat milk or unsweetened fruit juice and having it as a midmorning and midafternoon snack.

Soy products have always been a part of my nutrition programs because of their many benefits. Research studies have shown that an overabundance of the amino acid lysine increases the level of bad cholesterol in the body, while the amino acid arginine decreases it. Compared to animal protein, soy has a more favorable ratio of arginine to lysine. This lower ratio decreases the body's production of insulin and increases its production of glucagon. What this means is that eating soy every day helps you to shift your metabolism from fat storage to fat mobilization.

Soy products also help to lower the risk of coronary disease. And when used in conjunction with a properly balanced nutrition and aerobic exercise program, they are an important tool for lowering your body fat and cholesterol levels. Studies have shown that soy foods also lower the risk of hormone-related cancers.

In addition to soy-based powders, there are many delicious soy food products available, including soy burgers and hot dogs, many delicious varieties of tofu, soy cheeses, and soy milk. Soy products can be a nutritional mainstay for vegetarians faced by the challenge of getting sufficient protein in their daily diet.

When choosing other protein sources, always choose lean meats and low-fat dairy. First-choice protein sources include skim milk; fat-free cheese and cottage cheese; yogurt made from skim milk; 95 percent lean ground beef, turkey, or encased meats (e.g., sausage and bologna); white-meat, skinless chicken; white-meat tuna in water; egg whites; and nonfried fish and seafood.

According to the *American Journal of Clinical Nutrition,* eating fish daily decreases insulin levels, increases glucose production, lowers triglyceride (bad fat) production, and increases the level of HDL cholesterol (good cholesterol), reducing your risk of cardiovascular disease. For this reason, it is important to eat cold-water fish such as salmon, mackeral, and halibut at least twice a week.

The current RDA recommendation for protein is 0.8 grams per kilograms of body weight, but this does not provide enough for the dietary needs of individuals involved in regular exercise. Dr. E. C. Henley, who designed the food program in this chapter, suggests 60 to 100 grams of protein daily. If you want to know how many grams of protein are in a food source such as packaged meats or fish, nut butters, or soy products, simply read the label.

Getting your proper daily protein allotment is important for another reason. Based on a study of men between the ages of forty and seventy published in the *Journal of Clinical Endocrinology and Metabolism,* a diet with adequate amounts of protein helps stop the decrease in testosterone levels that many men experience as they age. The article goes on to say, "Diets low in protein lead to increases in sex hormone-binding globulin in older men, potentially reducing the availability of testosterone and causing loss of muscle mass, red cell mass and bone density."

Fats

In recent years, fats have gotten a bad reputation. But what most people do not realize is that by ingesting a daily diet of 25 percent of the *right* kinds of fat enables us to utilize dietary fat to help *burn* body fat. The reason for this is that all fats produce 9 calories of energy per gram and the body uses fats mostly as an energy source, along with glucose broken down from the digestion of carbohydrates.

There are two different groups of fat. The first, saturated fats, should be eaten only in limited amounts because they can clog your arteries, increasing your chances of heart disease. People who eat diets high in saturated fats also run a greater risk of developing some kinds of cancers. This types of fat is found in meat and dairy products such as beef, cheese, and butter.

The best kind of fat to include in your daily diet is monounsaturated fat, which is found in plant products such as vegetable oils, nuts, and avocados. Your body uses this type of fat to strengthen cell membranes, support nerve and hormone function, and produce hormonelike substances called prostaglandins, which have been linked to the prevention of heart disease and cancers.

Essential Fatty Acids Decrease Health Risks

Two kinds of unsaturated fats are necessary for your very survival. These are the essential fatty acids omega-6 (linoleic acid) and omega-3 (linolenic acid). Since your body cannot manufacture these fatty acids, they must be obtained from the foods you eat. Omega-6 is fairly common and is found in most of the vegetable oils sold in the grocery store. I suggest, however, that you try to buy your vegetable oils in health foods stores, if possible. Most typical grocery store oils, which are processed for mass distribution, are often filled with free radicals and bad fats called trans-fatty acids. Omega-3 is found in soy oil, walnut oil, flax oil, and canola oils and in dark green, leafy vegetables. I suggest that you purchase all oils in dark-colored green or amber bottles, since clear bottles tend to make the oils go rancid after a time due to chemical changes caused by exposure to sunlight.

It is especially important to make sure that you supplement your food plan with enough omega-3 fats, since the American diet is usually deficient in this nutrient. While the ideal ratio of omega-6 oil to omega-3 should be between 3:1 and 4:1, a recent study showed that for most people their level of omega-6 is 20 times their level of omega-3.

The benefits of ingesting the proper amount of unsaturated fats and essential fatty acids include:

- Lowering cholesterol levels
- Lowering high blood pressure
- Decreasing symptoms of heart palpitations and angina
- Preventing significantly the risk of heart attacks and strokes
- Decreasing the symptoms of multiple sclerosis
- Decreasing the pain and swelling of rheumatoid arthritis
- Correcting or markedly improving skin conditions such as psoriasis and eczema
- Lowering the risk of cancer

There are several other ways to increase the amount of essential fatty acids in your diet. For example, cold-water fish such as salmon, mackerel, and trout are rich sources of the essential fatty acid metabolites DHA (docosahexaenoic acid) and EPA (eicosapentaenoic acid). These have been shown to help lower blood pressure, improve cholesterol levels, and lower one's risk for cardiovascular disease. Aside from simply eating fish a minimum of twice per week, you can supplement your diet with omega-3 by taking fish oil capsules (taken with a meal), available at most pharmacies or health food stores.

Flax oil is another rich source of omega-3 and all essential fatty acids, which is why body builders mix it into their protein drinks so often. It is best taken not in capsules but in liquid form to make sure that it is fresh and of high quality. The next time you are fixing a green salad, try using a tablespoon of flax oil as a dressing, or half a tablespoon mixed with sunflower oil or a little vinegar. You may also lightly brush it over meat after it has been cooked.

Other acceptable oils or products containing oils include corn oil, Hellmann's Light Mayonnaise, Kraft Light Mayonnaise, Smart Balance Soft Spread (no trans-fatty acids), and unsaturated corn oil. Products such as Promise, Take Control, Fleischmann's Margarine, and I Can't Believe It's Not Butter! (spray, not solid) are excellent butter alternatives. If real butter is your only alternative when dining out, use it in moderation.

Fiber Is Important

Fiber is simply plant food that passes undigested through the small intestine. There are two basic types of fiber, insoluble and soluble. Insoluble fibers hold less water and include foods such as vegetables, most bran products, and whole grains. These types of foods provide bulk and help to normalize bowel movements. Soluble fibers hold up to forty times their weight in water, and include such foods as oats, any type of legume, beans, and psyllium. These kinds of foods provide the primary food source for friendly bacteria in the intestinal track. Not getting enough soluble fiber in your daily diet can lead to reduced growth of friendly bacteria, increased growth of unfriendly bacteria, constipation, and increased risk for colorectal cancer. Citrus fruits and apples, the most soluble fibers, hold 100 times their weight in water.

While the average person eats 16 to 17 grams of fiber per day, the National Cancer Institute recommends an average of 25 grams daily. A recent study by the American Dietetic Association, however, has caused the American Dietary Association to begin increasing its dietary recommendations of fiber. This study indicated that people with diabetes could significantly reduce their blood sugar by eating up to 50 grams of fiber per day. Other benefits of this high-fiber diet were an improved cholesterol level, lowering the participants' risk of heart disease, which is a major cause of death among people with diabetes.

A long-term study published recently in the *Journal of the American Medical Association* stated that eating a high-fiber diet also helps to fight obesity. On average, young adults who ate at least 21 grams of fiber per day gained eight pounds less over a ten-year period than those who ate the least amount of fiber. When you consider that a bowl of high-fiber cereal can contain up to 25 grams of fiber, it is not difficult to get sufficient fiber in your daily diet.

High-fiber foods include the following:

- Raw or lightly cooked vegetables.
- Cereals, rolls, and bread made from whole grain flour.
- Nuts, beans, peas, lentils, potatoes, and yams (with the skins on).
- Whole grains, such as whole wheat, brown rice, whole or rolled oats, buckwheat, amaranth, and brown rice.
- Raw fruits such as apples (with the skins on).
- Dried fruits such as raisins, apricots, dates, and prunes. (Buy organic dried fruits, since the drying process concentrates the level of fungicides and pesticides already present in nonorganic fruits.)

When you increase your daily intake of fiber, do it slowly to avoid discomfort and flatulence. Make sure to take a multivitamin, since fiber speeds digestion and might deplete the body of certain vitamins.

Assess Your Weight and Nutritional Habits

Now that you understand some of the nutritional basics, you are ready to take a questionnaire designed by E. C. Henley, Ph.D., R.D., an experienced nutrition researcher, professor, and counselor. This brief test will enable you to easily evaluate whether you are the right weight for your frame size and whether you are following a healthy food plan.

Nutritional Assessment Questionnaire

1. **Use the following guidelines to evaluate these statements:**

	Yes	No
I am at my ideal body weight.	☐	☐
I have an even distribution of fat in both my upper and my lower body.	☐	☐

Estimate Your Ideal Weight

If you are uncertain about your ideal body weight, you can estimate as follows:

Females: For the first 5 feet of height (60 inches) estimate 100 pounds. For each additional inch, add 5 pounds. So for a woman who is 5 feet 5 inches, an ideal weight would be about 125 pounds. Answer: _____.

Males: For the first 5 feet of height (60 inches) estimate 106 pounds. For each additional inch, add 5 pounds. So for a male who is 5 feet 10 inches, an ideal weight would be about 156 pounds. Answer: _____.

Estimate Your Frame Size

Your frame size will make a difference in estimating your ideal weight. Consider the figure calculated previously as the proper weight for a medium-size frame. If you have a small frame, your ideal weight could be about 10 percent less. If you have a large frame, your weight could be about 10 percent more.

Here's a rule of thumb for determining your frame size. Encircle the wrist of your opposing arm at the narrowest place with your thumb and index finger. If the two fingers overlap, your frame size is small. If they just meet, then your frame is medium. If there is a gap, your frame is on the large side. My frame size: _____.

Calculate Your Hip-to-Waist Ratio

The value of the hip measurement compared to the waist measurement is that it gives you some idea regarding the dangers associated with where your fat is stored. You have probably already heard that having a pear-shaped body is less dangerous than having an apple-shaped body. Fat that is stored around and above the waist results in a higher risk for diabetes and heart disease. The person with upper body fat distribution (the apple) loses fat quicker than the person with lower body fat distribution (the pear), but a smaller amount of fat stored above the waist is more dangerous than a larger amount of fat stored below the waist.

Here's how to determine your shape. Measure your waist at its narrowest circumference and your hips at their widest. Then divide your waist measurement by your hip measurement. For example, if you have a waist of 30 inches and a hip measurement of 42 inches, your hip-to-waist ratio is .71. For women, the preferred ratio is below .80 and for men below .95. Keep in mind that this measurement does not tell you anything about your total body weight or body composition. It just gives you an indication of *where* your excess fat is located and, therefore, your health risk relative to fat deposition.

My waist ratio is _____. My hip ratio is _____.
My hip-to-waist ratio is _____.

	Yes	No
2. **I look for ways to increase physical activity in my lifestyle.**	☐	☐
I regularly exercise thirty to sixty minutes per day.	☐	☐

Exercise lowers your risk for cancer, osteoporosis, heart disease, obesity, high blood pressure, and other diseases. Look for ways to incorporate more physical activity into your daily life such as taking the stairs; parking far away from your destination; and walking with your children, spouse, or dog. Bicycle to work if possible. Your exercise program should include aerobic, resistance, and flexibility exercises.

	Yes	No
3. **I am a nonsmoker.**	☐	☐
If I drink alcohol, I do so in moderation.	☐	☐

Quitting smoking is the single most important step you can take to safeguard your health. The American Institute of Cancer Research estimates that stopping smoking can drop cancer incidence by 30 percent. While drinking in moderation, especially red wine, has been linked to elevated HDL (good cholesterol) levels, drinking even one alcoholic beverage a day has been associated with breast cancer in women. The health benefits from red wine are attributed to the phytochemical resveratrol, which can also be found in grapes, grape juice, raisins, and peanuts.

	Yes	No

4. **I take care of my teeth, including daily flossing.** ☐ ☐
I eat at least two calcium-rich foods or take ☐ ☐
calcium supplements daily.

Good oral health is essential to enjoying a wide variety of foods. Loss of bone density can result not only in osteoporosis, but in loss of teeth as well. Sometimes it is difficult to obtain adequate amounts of calcium from your daily diet. Therefore, doctors recommend that you take calcium supplements. Since adequate amounts of vitamin D are required to enable your body to utilize calcium, be sure your supplement also contains vitamin D.

	Yes	No

5. **I avoid saturated and trans-fat in my daily diet,** ☐ ☐
eating mostly unsaturated fats.
(See page 117 for information on fats.)

	Yes	No

6. **I eat sufficient vegetables, including plant-based** ☐ ☐
proteins, and have two to three meatless meals
per week.

A diet comprised of significant amounts of vegetables and vegetable protein is associated with decreased risk of cancer, diabetes, heart disease, and obesity. If you currently eat animal protein (e.g., milk, meat, fowl, pork, eggs, cheese, and yogurt) at every meal, make a goal to have two to three meals per week that are vegetarian. Make sure, however, that these meals contain a sufficient amount of vegetable protein such as tofu or legumes, an appropriate amount of complex carbohydrates, and a sufficient amount of fats. Simply eating a big salad is not going to provide you with adequate nutritional fuel to maintain your metabolic needs and your energy levels. The American Institute of Cancer Research suggests that meat be used as a condiment instead of a main course. Be creative and experiment with beans, nuts, soy protein–based entrées, and whole grains.

	Yes	No

7. **I include seafood or fish in my diet one to two** ☐ ☐
times weekly.

Cold-water fish such as salmon and halibut contain omega-3 fatty acids, which promote a healthy heart and brain, and healthy joints and lungs. Even one to two servings per week is associated with lower rates of heart disease. If eating fish is not for you, consider taking fish oil supplements.

Yes   No

8. **I eat broccoli, cabbage, cauliflower, brussels sprouts, onions, garlic, or soy protein daily.**   ☐   ☐

These vegetables are especially important in lowering your risk for certain cancers. They contain antioxidant vitamins and phytochemicals that researchers are studying alone and in foods to determine their roles in cancer prevention. Soy protein plays a key role in the promotion of a healthy cardiovascular system. The FDA recommends 25 grams per day of soy protein for lowering the risk for heart disease.

Yes   No

9. **I eat at least two foods high in fiber each day.**   ☐   ☐

Fiber is important in maintaining a healthy gut and is useful in maintaining blood glucose levels within desirable levels. High-fiber diets satisfy our appetite and make us feel full, therefore aiding in weight maintenance. (See page 119 for more on fiber.)

Yes   No

10. **I eat red, yellow, and green fruits and vegetables daily.**   ☐   ☐

Red, yellow, and green fruits and vegetables are rich in the essential nutrients folic acid, vitamin C, and beta-carotene, as well as other important minerals and phytochemicals. Folic acid prevents birth defects and lowers blood homocysteine levels, a risk factor for heart disease. Potassium lowers the risk for hypertension. Current research on lycopenes, found in tomatoes (cooked are best), suggests that this substance plays a role in eye health and the prevention of cancer.

Yes   No

11. **I drink at least half an ounce of water per pound of body weight and two servings of tea daily.**   ☐   ☐

Most of your body is water. Even mild dehydration can lead to lethargy and constipation. Some evidence indicates that drinking adequate water may help prevent kidney stones and may be associated with a lower incidence of colon cancer. Tea, either green or black, contains polyphenols, which are powerful antioxidants. Polyphenols may lower the risk for cancer of the esophagus. In animal studies, they have been shown to lower the prevalence of skin tumors.

Yes   No

12. I confide in and often share meals with someone.   □   □

Data from survival and longevity studies suggest that having someone to socialize with during meals is an important component of
stress management and maintaining feelings of well-being.

Yes   No

13. I know my blood pressure and my blood lipid   □   □
     numbers.
     I practice appropriate eating and exercise   □   □
     behaviors.

Cardiovascular disease is the number one cause of death in the
United States in both men and women. Elevated blood pressure
causes kidney damage and places stress on arteries in the heart and
the brain, increasing the risk for both heart attacks and strokes.
There are effective dietary and pharmaceutical interventions for the
management of both elevated blood pressure and abnormal blood
lipids. Become familiar with your blood pressure and blood lipid
numbers—such as your HDL, LDL, total cholesterol, and triglyceride levels—and track them to monitor the success of your diet
and exercise program. If you need assistance in learning more
about your individual nutritional needs, or have severe health problems that can improve with proper nutrition, see a registered
dietitian.

Yes   No

14. I know the drug/drug and drug/nutrient inter-   □   □
     actions of any prescribed or over-the-counter
     medications I take.

Drug/drug interactions can be life threatening. Many times, com-
bining one medication with another can make a drug less effective
or more potent or can cause unwanted side effects. Many drugs
should be consumed either with foods or on an empty stomach.
Some medications taken with foods are either not absorbed well or,
conversely, may be absorbed in higher amounts than the manufac-
turer intended. Drug manufacturers have calculated the optimum
dosages for drugs when taken as prescribed. Check with a pharmacist about any special instructions related to drug, herbal supplement, or food interactions.

15. I eat slowly, enjoy meals without distractions,   □   □
  and leave food on my plate.

Eating slowly allows food to be fully absorbed and metabolized so that your brain can signal you when your hunger is satisfied. Research shows that when a person eats only the amount of food required to satisfy hunger, he or she will maintain a normal body weight. Distractions at meals increase the amount of food eaten, as they may dull your sensitivity as to whether or not your hunger is satisfied. Learn to listen to your body's signals and leave food on your plate when you are no longer hungry. Ironically, the major malnutrition problem in the United States is obesity, and this situation is increasing among children. Set an example for your children by eating slowly, enjoying meals without distractions, and leaving food on your plate.

Eat Healthfully with These Nutritional Guidelines

The following are Dr. E. C. Henley's guidelines for a healthy diet. They dovetail with the dietary recommendations for lowering the risk of cancer and heart disease recommended by organizations such as the National Heart Institute and the American College of Sports Medicine. In addition, these same guidelines are appropriate for managing weight, as serving sizes can simply be adjusted according to your individual caloric needs. Salt should be consumed in moderation, and foods containing simple sugars, honey, and syrup should be consumed within caloric needs and not at the expense of other recommended foods. Nutrient-dense foods such as complex carbohydrates and soy are especially important when one's calorie intake is limited, as in weight-loss diets or food plans for older individuals. *Bon appetit!*

Dietary Component	*Approximate Intake*
FOODS CONTAINING PROTEIN	60–100 grams protein
Vegetarian entrées several	(3–4 servings) daily
times per week	
At least 2 servings of fish per week	
25 grams soy protein daily	

Dietary Component	Approximate Intake
FOODS CONTAINING FIBER Beans, whole grains, vegetables, and fruits with skins and seeds	20–30 grams fiber daily
FRUITS Red grapes daily; dried cranberries 2–3 times per week; apples, berries, apricots, dried plums, melon, bananas, or citrus fruit daily	3–5 servings daily
VEGETABLES Garlic, cabbage, broccoli, spinach, onions, cauliflower, beans, peas, sweet potatoes, squash, greens, carrots, or 8–12 ounces tomato-based juice daily	3–5 servings daily
WHOLE-GRAIN FOODS Oatmeal, brown rice, whole wheat and rye breads/crackers, and high-fiber cereals daily	5–10 servings daily
FOODS CONTAINING FATS 3–4 servings of nuts per week Limit trans- and saturated fats Olives and avocados as desired within fat-calorie limit Season and sauté foods with olive oil	Limit fat intake to 20–30 percent of calories

Determine Your Caloric Needs

Before I show you some sample food programs incorporating Dr. E. C. Henley's recommendations, you need to determine how many calories your body actually needs by estimating your total daily caloric expenditure. This figure will include your resting metabolic rate (RMR)—the number of calories required for basic bodily processes such as tissue repair, brain function, blood circulation, and digestion—plus the number of calories burned during exercise and normal daily activity.

Step 1. If you are a woman, use the following formula to determine your RMR:

655 + (weight in kilograms × 9.6) + (height in cm × 1.8) − (age × 4.7)

To convert pounds to kilograms, divide them by 2.2. To convert inches to centimeters, multiply them by 2.5. For example, if you are a forty-year-old woman who weighs 125 pounds and is five feet six inches, you would divide 125 by 2.2 to get 56.8 kilograms. Then you would multiply 66 inches times 2.5 to get a height of 165 centimeters. You would then get out your calculator and plug those figures into the equation to get your RMR.

> Weight: 56.8 kilograms $\times$ 9.6 = 545.28
> Height: 165 cm $\times$ 1.8 = 297
> Age: 40 years old $\times$ 4.7 = 188
> Total: 655 + 545.28 + 297 − 188 = 1,309 calories (RMR)

If you are a man, use this formula to compute your RMR:

$$66 + (\text{weight in kg} \times 13.7) + (\text{height in cm} \times 5) - (\text{age} \times 6.8)$$

Since these formulas factor in gender, weight, height, and age, they are very precise and should be your preferred method for determining your RMR. However, if the math seems too much for you, a simple way to approximate your RMR is to multiply your body weight by 10. Using this formula, the 125-pound woman in the example has a resting metabolic rate of 1,250 calories.

Step 2. Since no one sits around all day without moving a muscle, you need to account for the calories burned during exercise and physical activity. A good rule of thumb is that a person will burn about two-thirds of his or her body weight in calories for every ten minutes of moderate cardiovascular exercise. So, our 125-pound woman would burn approximately 83.3 calories during every ten minutes of her cardio workout.

To calculate the actual number of calories you will need to support your daily level of activity, use the following criteria. If you are moderately active throughout your day, add about 40 to 60 percent of your resting metabolic rate. If your daily activities are sedentary—for example, if you sit at a desk most of the day— add only 20 percent of your resting metabolic rate. Let's look once again at our example of the 125-pound woman. If her RMR is 1,309 calories and she has a desk job, she would need to eat 1,309 + 261.8 = 1,570.8 calories daily to maintain her current weight. If she was moderately active, working out in the gym twice a week and doing aerobic exercises such as walking or bicycling five to six times per week, she would need to eat 1,309 + 523.6 = 1832.6 calories daily to maintain her current weight.

Keep in mind that these numbers are only an estimate. Several factors can affect an individual's metabolic rate, including age, genetics, certain medications, and body composition. Muscle is more metabolically active (burns more calories) than fat.

If you simply want to maintain your current weight, then you need to consume the number of calories you have determined as your total daily expenditure. If your goal is to lose weight, however, you'll need to cut back on your intake.

One pound of fat is equal to 3,500 calories. So, if you create a deficit of 500 calories a day, you should lose one pound each week. To accomplish this either increase your level of exercise and/or cut back on calories. Take care not to slash too many calories, though, because you don't want to deprive your body of the nutrients it needs. Consuming fewer than 1,200 calories per day is not recommended.

Following are four sample seven-day food plans designed by my nutritionist, Molly Kimball, based on the guidelines provided by Dr. Henley. These menus should give you an idea of how to properly apply these guidelines to a range of daily caloric requirements.

The 1,200-Calorie-a-Day Weekly Meal Plan

In this food plan, the caloric spread among proteins, fats, and carbohydrates is broken down in the following manner: 20 percent protein (60 grams), 25 percent fat (30 to 35 grams), and 55 percent carbohydrate (165 grams).

Day 1

BREAKFAST
- 4 egg-white omelette with diced onions, mushrooms, red and yellow peppers
- 1 slice 100 percent whole wheat toast
- 1 cup of tomato/vegetable juice

SNACK
>1 cup of soy yogurt topped with sliced peaches

LUNCH
>2–3 ounces baked halibut
>
>Stewed okra and tomatoes with onion, garlic, and ⅓ cup chickpeas prepared with 1 tsp olive oil

SNACK
>1 Tbsp soy nut butter on ½ whole grain bagel
>
>½ cup orange juice

DINNER
>Shrimp and vegetable curry: 2 ounces of shrimp (or tofu) with vegetables such as carrots, cauliflower, green beans, and onion with ginger, curry, and 1 Tbsp cashews
>
>1 cup of cooked bulgur

SNACK
>1 cup of skim milk blended with ice and 1 cup mixed berries, such as blueberries, blackberries, and strawberries

Day 2

BREAKFAST
>1 whole grain waffle topped with 1 Tbsp almond butter or soy nut butter
>
>½ cup sliced strawberries
>
>1 cup skim milk

SNACK
>½ cup of 100 percent grape juice
>
>4 whole grain crackers

LUNCH
>1 cup of tomato basil soup
>
>Veggie burger on whole grain bun
>
>Tossed mixed greens salad, with 1 Tbsp low-fat dressing

SNACK
>1 scoop of soy protein powder blended with water

DINNER
>2 ounces grilled teriyaki salmon
>
>1 cup spinach sautéed with 1 tsp olive oil, garlic, and onion
>
>⅓ cup basmati rice

SNACK
>1 cup of plain low-fat yogurt mixed with ½ cup blueberries

Day 3

BREAKFAST

Southwestern burrito: 2 egg whites, scrambled, sprinkle of low-fat cheddar, salsa, and ⅛ cup black beans rolled into a small whole wheat tortilla

1 cup of calcium-fortified rice milk

SNACK

2 small kiwis

1 ounce roasted soy nuts

LUNCH

Vegetable salad (zucchini, squash, eggplant, red and yellow peppers, grilled with 1 tsp olive oil) served over mixed greens

Top with 2 ounces of grilled shrimp and 1 Tbsp reduced fat herb vinaigrette dressing

½ baked sweet potato

SNACK

15 red grapes with 1 cup of low-fat yogurt

DINNER

1 cup of whole wheat pasta with 1 cup of tomato-based "meat" sauce, using veggie ground "meat" (or use 3 ounces of at least 93 percent lean ground beef).

Large Caesar salad with 1 Tbsp low-fat dressing

SNACK

Small grapefruit

Day 4

BREAKFAST

2 scoops soy protein powder blended with 8 ounces soy milk, ½ cup blackberries, 1 tsp psyllium, and ice

1 slice toasted oat bran bread

SNACK

7 dried apricots

1 mozzarella string cheese

LUNCH

1 cup of lentil soup

Mixed green salad with fresh veggies such as broccoli, cauliflower, tomatoes, and carrots topped with balsamic vinegar and 1 tsp olive oil

SNACK

1 cup of tomato/vegetable juice

6 almonds

DINNER
   2-ounce portion of swordfish baked in tomato-based sauce

   1 cup of couscous with diced vegetables

SNACK
   15 grapes

Day 5

BREAKFAST
   ¾ cup whole grain cereal (select a cereal with at least 5 grams of
      fiber per serving)

   Stir 1 scoop of soy protein powder into 1 cup of soy milk, and pour
      over cereal.

   Sprinkle with 1 Tbsp ground flaxseed

SNACK
   1 cup of honeydew melon

LUNCH
   1 cup of gazpacho soup

   Large spinach salad filled with 2 ounces grilled skinless chicken
      breast, 1 slice of avocado, ½ cup couscous, ⅓ cup black beans,
      and ½ cup grapes.

SNACK
   1 cup of low-fat yogurt

   1 cup of baby carrots

DINNER
   Kabobs made with 2 ounces shrimp, chicken, or very lean beef
      skewered with veggies such as onions, tomatoes, mushrooms,
      and red and yellow peppers

   Serve over ⅔ cup barley and brown rice pilaf

SNACK
   1 cup of sliced strawberries

Day 6

BREAKFAST
   1 cup cooked oatmeal with 1 scoop soy protein powder

   4 dried plums chopped into oatmeal

   1 carton of low-fat yogurt

SNACK
> ½ medium banana

LUNCH
> Roasted chicken salad: 2 ounces roasted, skinless chicken breast over mixed greens with cherry tomatoes, thinly sliced pears, ⅓ cup raspberries, and 1 Tbsp low-fat raspberry vinaigrette
>
> 5 whole grain crackers

SNACK
> 1 cup of tomato soup with 1 ounce of low-fat cheese

DINNER
> 3–4 ounces tofu stir-fried with portabella mushrooms, water chestnuts, carrots, onion, and garlic
>
> ½ cup tabbouleh

SNACK
> 1 cup of chocolate soy milk

Day 7

BREAKFAST
> ½ cup cooked bulgur mixed with 1 cup of soy milk
>
> Top with sliced apples, dried cranberries, and cinnamon

SNACK
> 1 cup of soy yogurt with 2 Tbsp raisins

LUNCH
> Fajitas: 2 ounces grilled shrimp, chicken, pork tenderloin, or tofu with onions; red, green, and yellow peppers; and 1 Tbsp guacamole

SNACK
> "Pizza": ½ whole wheat English muffin topped with tomato paste and 1 ounce of part-skim mozzarella

DINNER
> 2 ounces oven-roasted tuna with lime juice, fresh herbs, and 1 tsp olive oil
>
> Asparagus sautéed with onions
>
> Roasted sweet potato rounds seasoned with cinnamon, ground cloves, and ginger

SNACK
> 1 cup of sliced cantaloupe

The 1,500-Calorie-a-Day Sample Week Meal Plan

In this food plan, the caloric spread among proteins, fats, and carbohydrates is broken down in the following manner: 20 percent protein (75 grams), 25 percent fat (40 to 45 grams), 55 percent carbohydrate (205 grams).

Day 1

BREAKFAST

4 egg-white omelette with diced onion, mushrooms, red and yellow peppers, and 1 Tbsp diced olives

1 slice 100 percent whole wheat toast

1 small grapefruit

1 cup of tomato/vegetable juice

SNACK

1 cup of soy yogurt topped with sliced peaches

LUNCH

2–3 ounces baked halibut

Stewed okra and tomatoes with onion, garlic, and ⅔ cup chickpeas, prepared with 1 tsp olive oil

SNACK

1 Tbsp soy nut butter on ½ whole grain bagel

½ cup orange juice

DINNER

Shrimp and vegetable curry: 3 ounces of shrimp (or tofu), with vegetables such as carrots, cauliflower, green beans, and onion with ginger, curry, and 1 Tbsp cashews

1 cup of cooked bulgur

SNACK

1 cup of skim milk blended with ice and 1 cup mixed berries, such as blueberries, blackberries, and strawberries

Day 2

BREAKFAST

1 whole grain waffle topped with 1 Tbsp almond butter or soy nut butter

½ cup sliced strawberries

1 cup skim milk

SNACK

½ cup of 100 percent grape juice

4 whole grain crackers

LUNCH

1 cup of tomato basil soup

Veggie burger on whole grain bun with 1 Tbsp low-fat mayonnaise

Tossed mixed greens salad, with 1 Tbsp low-fat dressing

SNACK

1 scoop of soy protein powder blended with water

½ mango

DINNER

3 ounces grilled teriyaki salmon

1 cup spinach sautéed with 1 tsp olive oil, garlic, and onion

⅔ cup basmati rice

SNACK

1 CUP OF PLAIN LOW-FAT YOGURT MIXED WITH ½ CUP BLUEBERRIES

Day 3

BREAKFAST

Southwestern burrito: 2 egg whites, scrambled, sprinkle of low-fat
cheddar, salsa, and ⅛ cup black beans rolled into a small whole
wheat tortilla

½ cup of mango, cubed

1 cup of calcium-fortified rice milk

SNACK

2 small kiwis

1 ounce roasted soy nuts

LUNCH

Grilled vegetable salad (zucchini, squash, eggplant, red and yellow
peppers, grilled with 1 tsp olive oil) served over mixed greens

Top with 3 ounces of grilled shrimp, topped with 1 Tbsp reduced-fat
herb vinaigrette

1 baked sweet potato with 1 tsp butter

SNACK

15 RED GRAPES WITH 1 CUP OF LOW-FAT YOGURT

DINNER

1 cup of whole wheat pasta with 1 cup of tomato-based "meat" sauce,
using veggie ground "meat" (or 3 ounces of at least 93 percent lean
ground beef).

Large Caesar salad, with 1 Tbsp low-fat dressing

SNACK

Small grapefruit

Day 4

BREAKFAST

2 scoops soy protein powder blended with 8 ounces soy milk, ½ cup blackberries, 1 tsp psyllium, and ice

2 slices of toasted oat bran bread

SNACK

7 dried apricots

1 mozzarella string cheese

LUNCH

1 cup of lentil soup

Mixed greens salad with fresh veggies such as broccoli, cauliflower, tomatoes, and carrots, topped with balsamic vinegar and 1 tsp olive oil

SNACK

1 cup of tomato/vegetable juice

6 almonds

DINNER

3-ounce portion of swordfish, baked in tomato-based sauce

1 cup of couscous with diced vegetables and 1 Tbsp chopped walnuts

SNACK

30 grapes

Day 5

BREAKFAST

1½ cups whole grain cereal (select a cereal with at least 5 grams of fiber per serving) topped with ½ cup blueberries

Stir 1 scoop of soy protein powder into 1 cup of soy milk, and pour over cereal.

Sprinkle with 1 Tbsp ground flaxseed

SNACK

1 cup of honeydew melon

LUNCH

1 cup of gazpacho soup

Large spinach salad filled with 3 ounces grilled skinless chicken breast, 1 slice of avocado, ½ cup couscous, ⅓ cup black beans, and ½ cup grapes

SNACK

1 cup of low-fat yogurt

1 cup of baby carrots

DINNER

Kabobs made with 3 ounces shrimp, chicken, or very lean beef skewered with veggies such as onions, tomatoes, mushrooms, and red and yellow peppers

Serve over ⅔ cup barley and brown rice pilaf with 1 Tbsp pine nuts

SNACK

1 cup of sliced strawberries

Day 6

BREAKFAST

1 cup cooked oatmeal with 1 scoop soy protein powder

4 dried plums, chopped into oatmeal

1 carton of low-fat yogurt

SNACK

½ medium banana

LUNCH

Roasted chicken salad: 3 ounces roasted, skinless chicken breast over mixed greens, with cherry tomatoes, thinly sliced pears, ⅓ cup raspberries, and 1 Tbsp low-fat raspberry vinaigrette dressing

10 whole grain crackers

SNACK

1 cup of tomato soup with 1 ounce of low-fat cheese

DINNER

3–4 ounces tofu stir-fried in 1 tsp olive oil with portabella mushrooms, water chestnuts, carrots, onion, and garlic

½ cup tabbouleh

SNACK

1 cup of chocolate soy milk

1 apple

Day 7

BREAKFAST

1 cup cooked bulgur mixed with 1 cup of soy milk

Top with sliced apples, dried cranberries, and cinnamon

SNACK

1 cup of soy yogurt with 2 Tbsp raisins and 1 Tbsp flaxseed

½ cup of cranberry juice

LUNCH

Fajitas: 2 ounces grilled shrimp, chicken, pork tenderloin, or tofu filled with onions; red, green, and yellow peppers; and 1 Tbsp guacamole

SNACK
> "Pizza": ½ whole wheat English muffin topped with tomato paste and 1 ounce of part-skim mozzarella

DINNER
> 3 ounces oven-roasted tuna with lime juice, fresh herbs, and 1 tsp olive oil
>
> Asparagus sautéed with onions
>
> Roasted sweet potato rounds seasoned with cinnamon, ground cloves, and ginger

SNACK
> 1 cup of sliced cantaloupe

The 1,800-Calorie-a-Day Sample Week Meal Plan

In this food plan, the caloric spread among proteins, fats, and carbohydrates is broken down in the following manner: 20 percent protein (90 grams), 25 percent fat (50 grams), 55 percent carbohydrate (250 grams).

Day 1

BREAKFAST
> 4 egg-white omelette with diced onion, mushrooms, red and yellow peppers, and 1 Tbsp diced olives
>
> 2 slices 100 percent whole wheat toast with 1 tsp of yogurt spread
>
> 1 small grapefruit
>
> 1 cup of tomato/vegetable juice

SNACK
> 1 cup of soy yogurt topped with sliced peaches

LUNCH
> 3 ounces baked halibut
>
> Stewed okra and tomatoes with onion, garlic, and ⅔ cup chickpeas, prepared with 1 tsp olive oil
>
> Small baked apple
>
> 1 cup of soy milk

SNACK
> 1 Tbsp soy nut butter on ½ whole grain bagel
>
> ½ cup orange juice

DINNER

 Shrimp and vegetable curry: 3 ounces of shrimp (or tofu), with
  vegetables such as carrots, cauliflower, green beans, and onion
  with ginger, curry, and 1 Tbsp cashews

 1 cup of cooked bulgur

SNACK

 1 cup of skim milk blended with ice and 1 cup mixed berries,
  such as blueberries, blackberries, and strawberries

Day 2

BREAKFAST

 2 whole grain waffles topped with 1 Tbsp almond butter or
  soy nut butter

 ½ cup sliced strawberries

 1 cup skim milk

SNACK

 ½ cup of 100 percent grape juice

 4 whole grain crackers

LUNCH

 1 cup of tomato basil soup

 Veggie burger on whole grain bun

 Top with 1 slice of mozzarella cheese and 1 tbsp light mayonnaise

 Tossed mixed greens salad, with 1 Tbsp low-fat dressing

SNACK

 1 scoop of soy protein powder blended with 1 cup of skim milk

 ½ mango

DINNER

 3 ounces grilled teriyaki salmon with ½ cup diced pineapple

 1 cup spinach sautéed with 1 tsp olive oil, garlic, and onion

 ⅔ cup basmati rice

SNACK

 1 cup of plain low-fat yogurt mixed with ½ cup blueberries

Day 3

BREAKFAST

 Southwestern burrito: 1 egg plus 2 egg whites, scrambled, sprinkle of
  low-fat cheddar, salsa, ⅛ avocado, and ⅓ cup black beans rolled into
  2 small whole wheat tortillas

 ½ cup of mango, cubed

 1 cup of calcium-fortified rice milk

SNACK

 2 small kiwis

 1 ounce roasted soy nuts

LUNCH
> Grilled vegetable salad (zucchini, squash, eggplant, red and yellow peppers, grilled with 1 tsp olive oil) served over mixed greens
>
> Top with 3 ounces of grilled shrimp, topped with 1 Tbsp reduced-fat herb vinaigrette
>
> 1 baked sweet potato with 1 tsp butter

SNACK
> 30 red grapes with 1 cup of low-fat yogurt

DINNER
> 1 cup of whole wheat pasta with 1 cup of tomato-based "meat" sauce, using veggie ground "meat" (or 3 ounces of 93 percent lean ground beef).
>
> Large Caesar salad, with 1 Tbsp low-fat dressing

SNACK
> Small grapefruit
>
> 1 cup of vanilla soy milk

Day 4

BREAKFAST
> 2 scoops soy protein powder blended with 8 ounces soy milk, ½ cup blackberries, 1 tsp psyllium, and ice
>
> 2 slices of toasted oat bran bread

SNACK
> 7 dried apricots
>
> 1 mozzarella string cheese
>
> 1 small bran muffin

LUNCH
> 1 cup of lentil soup
>
> Mixed greens salad with fresh veggies such as broccoli, cauliflower, tomatoes, and carrots, topped with 2 Tbsp golden raisins, balsamic vinegar and 2 tsp olive oil
>
> 1 carton of low-fat yogurt

SNACK
> 1 cup of tomato/vegetable juice
>
> 6 almonds

DINNER
> 4-ounce portion of swordfish, baked in tomato-based sauce
>
> 1 cup of couscous with diced vegetables and 1 Tbsp chopped walnuts

SNACK
> 30 grapes

Day 5

BREAKFAST

> 1½ cups whole grain cereal (select a cereal with at least 5 grams of fiber per serving) topped with ½ cup blueberries
>
> Stir 1 scoop of soy protein powder into 1 cup of soy milk, and pour over cereal.
>
> Sprinkle with 1 Tbsp ground flaxseed

SNACK

> 1 cup of honeydew melon

LUNCH

> 1 cup of gazpacho soup
>
> Large spinach salad filled with 3 ounces grilled skinless chicken breast, 1 slice of avocado, ½ cup couscous, ⅛ cup black beans, and ½ cup grapes

SNACK

> 1 cup of low-fat yogurt mixed with 10 cherries and ¼ cup dry rolled oats
>
> 1 cup of baby carrots

DINNER

> Kabobs made with 3 ounces shrimp, chicken, or very lean beef skewered with veggies such as onions, tomatoes, mushrooms, red and yellow peppers
>
> Serve over ⅔ cup barley and brown rice pilaf, with 1 Tbsp pine nuts

SNACK

> 1 cup of sliced strawberries

Day 6

BREAKFAST

> 1 cup cooked oatmeal with 1 scoop soy protein powder
>
> 4 dried plums, chopped into oatmeal
>
> 1 carton of low-fat yogurt

SNACK

> 1 slice of 100 percent whole wheat bread topped with 1 Tbsp peanut butter and ½ medium banana

LUNCH

> Roasted chicken salad: 3 ounces roasted, skinless chicken breast over mixed greens, with cherry tomatoes, thinly sliced pears, ⅓ cup raspberries, and 1 Tbsp low-fat raspberry vinaigrette dressing
>
> 10 whole grain crackers

SNACK

> 1 cup of tomato soup with 1 ounce of low-fat cheese

DINNER
>3–4 ounces tofu stir-fried in 1 tsp olive oil with portabella mushrooms, water chestnuts, carrots, onion, and garlic
>
>½ cup tabbouleh

SNACK
>1 cup of chocolate soy milk
>
>1 apple

Day 7

BREAKFAST
>1 cup cooked bulgur mixed with 1 cup of soy milk
>
>Top with sliced apples, dried cranberries, and cinnamon
>
>½ cup of 100 percent grape juice

SNACK
>1 cup of soy yogurt with 2 Tbsp raisins and 1 Tbsp flaxseeds
>
>½ cup of cranberry juice

LUNCH
>Fajitas: 3 ounces grilled shrimp, chicken, pork tenderloin, or tofu and ⅓ cup black beans filled with onions; red, green, and yellow peppers; and 1 Tbsp guacamole

SNACK
>"Pizza": ½ whole wheat English muffin topped with tomato paste and 1 ounce of part-skim mozzarella
>
>1 cup of skim milk

DINNER
>3 ounces oven-roasted tuna with lime juice, fresh herbs, and 1 tsp olive oil
>
>Asparagus sautéed with onions and 1 Tbsp sliced almonds
>
>Roasted sweet potato rounds seasoned with cinnamon, ground cloves, and ginger

SNACK
>1 cup of sliced cantaloupe

The 2,000-Calorie-a-Day Sample Week Meal Plan

In this food plan, the caloric spread among proteins, fats, and carbohydrates is broken down in the following manner: 20 percent protein (100 grams), 25 percent fat (55 grams), 55 percent carbohydrate (275 grams).

Day 1

BREAKFAST

> 4 egg-white omelette with diced onion, mushrooms, red and yellow peppers, and 1 Tbsp diced olives
>
> Top with 1 slice of part-skim mozzarella cheese
>
> 2 slices 100 percent whole wheat toast with 1 tsp of yogurt spread
>
> 1 small grapefruit
>
> 1 cup of tomato/vegetable juice

SNACK

> 1 cup of soy yogurt topped with sliced peaches

LUNCH

> 3 ounces baked halibut
>
> Stewed okra and tomatoes with onion, garlic, and ⅔ cup chickpeas, prepared with 1 tsp olive oil
>
> 1 whole wheat pita, toasted
>
> Small baked apple
>
> 1 cup of soy milk

SNACK

> 1 Tbsp soy nut butter on ½ whole grain bagel
>
> ½ cup orange juice

DINNER

> Shrimp and vegetable curry: 3 ounces of shrimp (or tofu), with vegetables such as carrots, cauliflower, green beans, and onion with ginger, curry, and 1 Tbsp cashews
>
> 1 cup of cooked bulgur

SNACK

> 1 cup of skim milk blended with ice and 1 cup mixed berries, such as blueberries, blackberries, and strawberries

Day 2

BREAKFAST

> 2 whole grain waffles topped with 1 Tbsp almond butter or soy nut butter
>
> ½ cup sliced strawberries
>
> 1 cup skim milk

SNACK

> ½ cup of 100 percent grape juice
>
> 4 whole grain crackers topped with 2 Tbsp hummus

LUNCH

> 1 cup of tomato basil soup

Veggie burger on whole grain bun

Top with 1 slice of mozzarella cheese and 1 Tbsp light mayonnaise

Tossed mixed greens salad, with 1 Tbsp low-fat dressing

SNACK

1 scoop of soy protein powder blended with 1 cup of skim milk

Pour over 1½ cups of cereal

½ mango

DINNER

4 ounces grilled teriyaki salmon with ½ cup diced pineapple

1 cup spinach sautéed with 1 tsp olive oil, garlic, and onion

⅔ cup basmati rice

SNACK

1 cup of plain low-fat yogurt mixed with ½ cup blueberries

Day 3

BREAKFAST

Southwestern burrito: 1 egg plus 2 egg whites, scrambled, sprinkle of low-fat cheddar, salsa, ⅛ avocado, and ⅓ cup black beans rolled into 2 small whole wheat tortillas

½ cup of mango, cubed

1 cup of calcium-fortified rice milk

SNACK

2 small kiwis

1 ounce roasted soy nuts

½ cup of apple juice

LUNCH

Grilled vegetable salad (zucchini, squash, eggplant, red and yellow peppers, grilled with 1 tsp olive oil) over mixed greens

Top with 3 ounces of grilled shrimp, topped with 1 Tbsp reduced-fat herb vinaigrette

1 baked sweet potato with 1 tsp butter

SNACK

30 red grapes

1 cup of low-fat yogurt topped with ¾ cup of whole grain cereal

DINNER

1 cup of whole wheat pasta with 1 cup of tomato-based "meat" sauce, using veggie "ground meat" (or 3 ounces of at least 93 percent lean ground beef).

Large Caesar salad, with 1 tbsp lowfat dressing

SNACK

Small grapefruit

1 cup of vanilla soy milk with 1 scoop of soy protein powder

3 cups of air-popped popcorn, no oils/butters added

Day 4

BREAKFAST

2 scoops soy protein powder blended with 8 ounces soy milk, ½ cup blackberries, 1 tsp psyllium, and ice

2 slices of toasted oat bran bread

SNACK

7 dried apricots

1 mozzarella string cheese

1 small bran muffin

LUNCH

1 cup of lentil soup

Mixed greens salad with fresh veggies such as broccoli, cauliflower, tomatoes, and carrots, topped with 2 Tbsp golden raisins, balsamic vinegar and 2 tsp olive oil

1 carton of low-fat yogurt

SNACK

1 cup of tomato/vegetable juice

1 cup of steamed edamame, in pods

6 almonds

DINNER

4-ounce portion of swordfish, baked in tomato-based sauce

1 cup of couscous with diced vegetables and 1 Tbsp chopped walnuts

SNACK

30 grapes over ¼ cup of low-fat cottage cheese, with 1 Tbsp ground flaxseed

Day 5

BREAKFAST

1½ cups whole grain cereal (select a cereal with at least 5 grams of fiber per serving) topped with ½ cup blueberries

Stir 1 scoop of soy protein powder into 1 cup of soy milk, and pour over cereal.

Sprinkle with 1 Tbsp ground flaxseed

1 slice of sprouted grain bread with 1 tsp yogurt spread

SNACK

1 cup of honeydew melon

3 sheets of Wasa fiber rye crackers with 1 Tbsp almond butter

LUNCH

>   1 cup of gazpacho soup
>
>   Large spinach salad filled with 3 ounces grilled skinless chicken
>   breast, 1 slice of avocado, ½ cup couscous, ⅛ cup black beans,
>   and ½ cup grapes

SNACK

>   1 cup of low-fat yogurt mixed with 10 cherries and ¼ cup dry
>   rolled oats
>
>   1 cup of baby carrots

DINNER

>   Kabobs made with 3 ounces shrimp, chicken, or very lean beef
>   skewered with veggies such as onions, tomatoes, mushrooms,
>   red and yellow peppers
>
>   Serve over ⅔ cup barley and brown rice pilaf, with 1 Tbsp pine nuts

SNACK

>   Parfait: 1 cup of sliced strawberries layered with 1 cup of plain
>   low-fat yogurt

Day 6

BREAKFAST

>   1 cup cooked oatmeal with 1 scoop soy protein powder
>
>   4 dried plums, chopped into oatmeal
>
>   1 carton of low-fat yogurt

SNACK

>   1 Tbsp peanut butter, 1 Tbsp wheat germ, 1 Tbsp honey,
>   and ½ medium banana
>
>   On 2 slices of 100 percent whole grain bread

LUNCH

>   Roasted chicken salad
>
>   3 ounces roasted, skinless chicken breast over mixed greens, with
>   cherry tomatoes, thinly sliced pears, ⅛ cup raspberries, and 1 Tbsp
>   low-fat raspberry vinaigrette
>
>   10 whole grain crackers

SNACK

>   1 cup of tomato soup with 1 ounce of low-fat cheese

DINNER

>   4–6 ounces tofu stir-fried in 1 tsp olive oil with portabella mushrooms,
>   water chestnuts, carrots, onion, and garlic
>
>   ½ cup tabbouleh

SNACK

>   1 cup of chocolate soy milk
>
>   1 apple

Day 7

BREAKFAST

    1 cup cooked bulgur mixed with 1 cup of soy milk

    Top with sliced apples, dried cranberries, and cinnamon

    ½ cup of 100 percent grape juice

SNACK

    1 cup of soy yogurt with 2 Tbsp raisins and 1 Tbsp flaxseed

    ½ cup of cranberry juice

LUNCH

    Fajitas: 3 ounces grilled shrimp, chicken, pork tenderloin, or tofu
        and ⅔ cup of black beans filled with onions; red, green, and yellow
        peppers; and 1 Tbsp guacamole

SNACK

    "Pizza": Whole wheat English muffin topped with tomato paste and
        1 ounce of part-skim mozzarella

    1 cup of skim milk

DINNER

    4 ounces oven-roasted tuna with lime juice, fresh herbs, and 1 tsp
        olive oil

    Asparagus sautéed with onions and 1 Tbsp sliced almonds

    Roasted sweet potato rounds seasoned with cinnamon, ground cloves,
        and ginger

SNACK

    1½ cups fresh fruit mix (cantaloupe, honeydew, papaya, pineapple)

The Wellness Organizer

One of the tools that I give to clients is a Wellness Organizer. This system is a variation on the "Skinny Box" initially developed by Hal C. Becker, Ph.D., my field faculty adviser in graduate school. This Wellness Organizer has twelve categories designed to enhance your overall wellness profile. The thousands of clients I have worked with are evidence that if a person uses the Wellness Organizer to its fullest extent, he or she will lose a minimum of two pounds of fat per week. The behavioral modification categories included in the Wellness Organizer are as follows:

Category 1: Calories in the kitchen. Place all food in the kitchen. Eating only in a designated area such as the kitchen or dining room will help you to stop eating snacks while watching TV or relaxing in another part of the house.

Category 2: Four to five per day. Eat at least four to five small meals daily. Eating meals and planned snacks will stabilize your insulin level and mobilize body fat to be burned during your exercise sessions.

Category 3: Eat less. By putting less food on your plate, you remove the temptation to overeat. Put one bite from your plate back into the serving dish before you sit down to eat.

Category 4: One-two stop. Eat two morsels of food with proper chewing, then stop eating before the third bite and put your fork down. If you consume your meal in less than twenty minutes, your brain does not have a chance to get the message that you are being adequately nourished and you will feel hungry and frustrated. By eating slowly, you are sending a signal to the hypothalmus, the brain's thermostat, that food is in your system.

Category 5: Eight's too late. When you eat is also important. Never eat anything heavy later than 8:00 P.M. because eating late does not allow your body time to utilize the calories. If you are hungry after eight, I suggest that you mix a tablespoon of soy protein powder into juice or water to increase your metabolic rate. If you must eat after eight because of your busy schedule, try to allow two hours between your last meal and bedtime.

Category 6: No junk food between. Eating junk food calories between meals can add unwanted excess fat. Only eat appropriate snacks between meals.

Category 7: Never when upset. It is always best not to eat when under any type of stress, since you are not aware of what or of how much you are consuming when distracted by a stressor. Many people also eat the wrong types of foods—"comfort foods" such as desserts and pizza—when stressed.

Category 8: Proper rest. Obtaining seven to eight hours of sleep per night is a very important part of any successful nutritional or stress reduction program. Night is your body's time for recuperation. Your kidneys also function best in a prone position. Make sure you are sound asleep before midnight to achieve the deep REM sleep state that truly relaxes your body and allows it to recuperate.

Category 9: Drink enough water. To give you the proper hydration level to keep your kidneys working properly and your body's internal insulatory thermostat working properly so that you do not hoard fat, you should drink between one-half to one ounce of water per pound of body weight per day. Water is one of your greatest allies in the business of weight loss.

Category 10: Aerobic zone. You need to exercise in your aerobic fat-burning zone on a regular basis. (See chapter 13 for my complete exercise program.)

Category 11: Brush your teeth. Brushing your teeth after each meal provides a sense of closure, changes the chemistry in your mouth, and reduces the urge to go back to the table and overeat.

Category 12: Visualize. Use some form of meditation to help reduce stress and to visualize your weight loss and exercise goals.

How to Score the Wellness Organizer

Review each of the twelve categories daily and give yourself one point for each one that you achieve. A perfect daily score is 12 and a perfect weekly score is 84. Don't be discouraged, however, if your first few weeks are less than perfect. Think of this as a tool to help you see which areas you are strong in and which you need to work on and keep improving. Remember, you will only lose two pounds per week if you follow each step faithfully.

I have included the following chart that you can photocopy to use over and over again.

If you allow the nutritional program in this chapter to become a part of your lifestyle, you will never again have to experience the frustration, hunger, and disappointments of fad diets that do not deliver on their promises to help you take off weight and keep it off. If you follow my stress management and exercise programs coupled with proper nutrition, you will be guaranteed not only to lose unhealthy fat and gain lean muscle, but also consistently to experience greater health, vitality, performance levels, and longevity than you have ever dreamed possible.

WELLNESS ORGANIZER

	Sunday	Monday	Tuesday	Wednesday	Thursday	Friday	Saturday	Weekly totals
1. Calories in the kitchen								
2. Four to five per day								
3. Eat less								
4. One-two stop								
5. Eight's too late								
6. No junk food between								
7. Never when upset								
8. Proper rest								
9. Drink enough water								
10. Aerobic zone								
11. Brush your teeth								
12. Visualize								
Daily totals								

11

Eleven Life-Transforming Benefits of Exercise

Professional athletes spend a great deal of money, time, and effort on improving the quality of their performance. If they don't perform well, they know they are out of the game, so they train to be strong, fast, and competitive. In short, they are playing to win.

If professional athletes work so hard at ensuring that they are at the top of their form in careers that may last only a few years or a decade, how much more should you pay attention to how well *you* perform? You must maintain and improve your levels of performance in a career lasting *forty years*. How much harder should you work to make sure that you preserve your health, lower your risk factors, and keep yourself focused?

Eleven Reasons Why Exercise Should Be a Part of Your Lifestyle

While most people would agree that exercise is important, few really understand the immense benefits one derives from a good workout program. Studies have shown that even as few as ten minutes a day of aerobic activities such as walking can have positive effects on one's health. Let's take a moment to examine ten benefits you will receive from a program of consistent and appropriate exercise.

Benefit 1: Improve Your Cardiovascular Fitness

A recent study published in the journal *Circulation* showed that exercise can improve the cardiovascular system even if a person hasn't exercised in years. This study involved men in their fifties who participated in a training program that included walking, jogging, and/or cycling. At the end of six months, they were exercising an average of 4.5 hours a week and had turned back their cardiovascular fitness clock by decades. As stated in the study, "An endurance program using a relatively modest intensity of training was able to return the group to the levels of aerobic power they had 30 years ago."

Although heart disease is the number one killer in the United States, as I've said, it is also the easiest disease to either avoid or improve. Proper and consistent exercise that includes a significant cardiovascular component is one of the most effective tools for fighting this disease.

Benefit 2: Lower Your Resting Heart Rate

Your heart beats an average of 100,000 times per day. Over an average life span of seventy-eight years, your blood will have traveled throughout your entire body via your circulatory system a total of two-and-a-half billion times. It stands to reason that the person who is physically conditioned and has a slower resting heartbeat will be able to maintain his or her optimum performance level for much longer than someone whose resting heartbeat is high. For example, while the average resting heartbeat is sixty to seventy beats per minute for a man and seventy to eighty beats per minute for a woman, my resting heartbeat is only thirty-nine beats per minute because I am highly aerobically conditioned.

You can lower your resting heartbeat starting at any age. One sixty-seven-year-old client named George in my PEP program has developed a remarkable level of fitness over the last two years. While George's resting heart rate was already in the lower range for a man his age, sixty-six to seventy-two beats per minute, it has now dropped into the range of fifty to sixty-four beats. The remarkable thing about him, however, is his recovery rate—the amount of time that it takes for his heartbeat to slow after intense exercise. After exercising at his target heart rate, George's heartbeat drops back under 90 bpm in thirty seconds flat. Many younger men's and women's hearts cannot do this.

Benefit 3: Improve Your Mood

Tensions, worries, depression, and mood swings undermine one's work performance, personal life, and ability to feel motivated and in control. Research has shown that people who make exercise a regular part of their lifestyle experience improvement in moods and a greater ability to handle the worries of daily life. One reason is the kind of chemicals released into the bloodstream during exercise. Studies that compare the body chemistry of joggers and those who do other types of exercise to the body chemistry of sedentary individuals have shown that a greater percentage of mood-elevating substances such as endorphins is found in the bloodstream of those who are regularly involved in cardiovascular fitness activities. Exercise improves one's mental outlook and self-esteem, helps to release pent-up feelings, and alleviates the symptoms of moderate depression.

Benefit 4: Relieve Your Stress

People who live with high levels of stress will be amazed at how effectively exercise combats stress. Stress is a killer because it undermines almost every system in the body, from the cardiovascular system to the immune system. Since I work with so many professionals whose jobs come with an unavoidable stress component, I am always gratified to see how greatly my Pro Circuit Exercise Program improves their ability to handle stress.

One remarkable story of someone who increased his ability to deal with stress through the program is Deputy Chief Marlon Defillo of the New Orleans Police Department. Few professionals experience the level or type of stress that police officers do because these men and women deal, literally, with life and death situations. A recent study done at the University College of the Fraser Valley in Abbotsford, British Columbia, demonstrated that police officers experience high levels of stress during the full twenty-four hours of their day. They experience anticipatory stress at the beginning of their work shifts, psychosocial stress on the job, and the highest levels of stress prior to answering calls for on-site assistance. Nor does this stress dissipate by the end of their shift.

When Deputy Chief Defillo began my Pro Circuit Program he was only thirty-seven, a very young man. But he was already experiencing serious health problems from his job-related stress. He suffered from such severe headaches that he was taking up to twelve painkillers a day, anything from Advil to Aleve. Sometimes he developed migraines that lasted from two to three days, causing him severe nausea. He was convinced that his headaches were stress induced, caused by the violence of the crime scenes he had to respond to as part of his job. For the last ten years he had investigated homicides and, prior to that, child abuse cases and crime scenes where children had been murdered by their parents. Deputy Chief Defillo stated:

> My whole professional life centered around other folks' grief and despair. I needed something to reduce stress. There were days when I just was not functional. I would get to work and just have to sit here. I couldn't drive. I couldn't leave. I had to find some outlet. When I got into Mackie's program it all went away. I didn't have to take the headache pills anymore. Everything changed because my whole management of stress changed through the workout program. I didn't suffer with those headaches any longer. I was able to manage stress and be functional at work and at home. The program has become such a regime for me. If I don't work out I feel like I'm missing something.

Not only did the Pro Circuit reduce Deputy Chief Defillo's stress and rid him of his chronic headaches, but his weight also dropped from 248 pounds to 217 pounds, he went from 25 percent body fat to 12 percent, and his waistline decreased from forty inches to thirty-four inches. This last figure is especially significant, considering that a waistline of forty inches or more in a man is a sure indicator of severe risk for illnesses such as type 2 diabetes and cardiovascular disease.

Benefit 5: Lose Fat, Not Lean Muscle, When Dieting

When people try to lose weight without exercising, they run the risk of losing lean tissue. Ironically, you may end up *worse off* at the end of your diet than when you started, with a lower scale weight but with a higher percentage of body fat (metabolically inactive tissue). *Just going on a diet is not enough.* Only proper nutrition coupled with appropriate exercise will insure that you lose fat while building lean muscle. What's more, people who continue to exercise after weight loss will be much more likely to maintain their new weight than people who stop exercising when their diet is over.

Benefit 6: Increase Your Metabolic Rate

According to Dr. Michael T. Murray and Joseph E. Pizzorno in their book *The Encyclopedia of Natural Medicine,* physical inactivity is the reason why so many people are overweight. Low activity levels contribute to the slowing of one's metabolic rate. Exercise, on the other hand, increases your metabolic rate, your ability to utilize calories more efficiently and burn fat. Since metabolically active muscle tissue is the primary user of fat calories in the body, the more lean muscle you can develop through exercise and proper nutrition, the more efficient your body can become as a fat-burning machine.

A client of mine, Amy, changed from a job that required a lot of standing and walking to one where she sat at a desk all day long. Within four years, she had gained twenty pounds. She originally came to me with the goal of simply losing weight by getting into a good nutritional program. But when she discovered that her body fat was 37 percent, making her, by definition, obese, she decided that she needed to start exercising as well. Over the last year, she's not only lost twenty-five pounds, more than she originally planned, but she dropped her body fat percentage by 13 points to a much healthier 24 percent. She's carrying around less metabolically inactive tissue and more lean muscle.

Benefit 7: Increase Your Overall Health Profile

According to a recent article released by the American College of Sports Medicine, which cross-referenced results from worldwide studies conducted by the University of Oulu, Finland; the University of Vermont; the Mayo Clinic; and other studies done in England, Belgium, and Canada, people who exercise regularly experience a wide range of health benefits, regardless of age or gender. These include:

- Lowering of total cholesterol
- Raising of one's level of HDL (good cholesterol)
- Decrease in blood pressure and hypertension
- Decrease in insulin sensitivity
- Prevention of type 2 diabetes and lower mortality rates in those with this disease
- Lowering of both incidence and mortality from all forms of coronary heart disease
- Improved coagulation of the blood
- Decrease in one's risk for colon cancer

Benefit 8: Decrease Your Back and Joint Pain

An alarming 50 percent of people over the age of thirty suffer from pain in at least one joint and from low back pain. These conditions have been brought on by a variety of causes, including sports injuries, overuse of joints in activities such as excessive jogging, strain on the joints and back from obesity, a sedentary lifestyle, and poor posture caused by the weakening of the muscles in the core area of the body.

If done incorrectly and at too great a level of intensity, exercise can have detrimental effects on back and joint pain. But if done correctly and under a doctor's supervision, exercise can decrease lower back pain significantly by strengthening the core area of the body. It can also lessen the effects of osteoarthritis by increasing joint flexibility and range of motion.

A colleague of mine, Dr. Mike Wilson, tells all of his clients with chronic lower back pain to get into a good program of exercises for the core area of the body. The Pro Circuit Exercise Program in this book will do wonders toward relieving your lower back pain. If you feel the need for further back-strengthening exercises, I suggest my book *Lose Your Love Handles,* in which I offer a program designed solely for strengthening this core area of the body—the abdominals and the lower back.

Benefit 9: Avoid or Decrease Loss of Bone Density and Muscle Mass

Most people believe that a significant loss of muscle mass (sarcopenia) and bone density is inevitable as one ages, leading to decreased strength, mobility, and flexibility. This is not so. According to a recent article published in the *Journal of the American Academy of Orthopaedic Surgeons,* most age-related changes in muscle and bone can be reversed through an appropriate exercise program incorporating both aerobic and resistance/strength training (working with weights or objects one has to push against).

Individuals suffering from sarcopenia and bone loss experience a significant decrease in energy levels and strength. A special issue of *Newsweek* focusing on longevity reported how a seventy-six-year-old woman, Barbara, was finding it more and more difficult to do simple things such as getting up out of her favorite easy chair. Bending over to make her bed was so painful that she had to get down on her knees to do so. At 140 pounds, Barbara was not overweight, but her fat to lean muscle ratio was extremely high. She described herself as "mostly flab and mush." This is not surprising, since people who lose muscle as they age also gain body fat—and most of us do. Remember, a greater body fat to lean muscle ratio also means a less efficient metabolism, since fat is not metabolically active. It just sits there on your body, pulling you down.

When her doctor told her that she was suffering from low bone density as well, Barbara knew she had to do something to help herself. She enrolled in a study at Oregon State University that was researching the effects of exercise on bone density in women over fifty. The study was exploring the hypothesis that gradually reintroducing women to exercise would increase bone density and muscle mass. The women began by wearing weighted vests and practicing everyday movements such as standing up, walking, and stepping from side to side. They gradually moved on to more strenuous activities, such as four-inch high jumps. Once Barbara began to gain back some of her lost bone and muscle mass, she started exercising regularly with her husband and now says she is more fit at eighty-one than she was at forty. "I can't describe the feeling—it's a sense of being stronger and more accomplished and less afraid. You can't just give up and go downhill. Life is just too precious."

It used to be that men and women past the age of fifty were expected to be flabby. For many, that attitude is changing as they discover that even a moderate amount of exercise makes muscles stronger and joints more flexible and arrests the loss of bone density (a problem in aging men as well as women). In fact, the *Canadian Journal of Applied Physiology* reports that studies on sarcopenia unequivocally show that older muscle tissue has the same, if not an even greater capacity, to respond to a vigorous bout of resistance exercise than younger muscle does.

Women: Defeat Osteoporosis through Exercise

Of special interest to women is the fact that osteoporosis can be either prevented or slowed by the consistent practice of a good resistance exercise program. In fact, the older a woman gets, the more important exercise becomes to her musculoskeletal health and strength. Think how many women you know who can barely get around in their seventies, eighties, and nineties. Since women live longer than men, it is especially important for them to keep relatively fit so that their quality of life does not degrade in their later years.

Benefit 10: Decrease the Severity of Physical Injury

Exercise helps to prevent injury in people of all ages by increasing flexibility, strength, balance, and the overall health of the musculoskeletal system. We all know that breaking a bone can be serious after the age of sixty because of slower healing processes. People who exercise are much more likely to have breaks that heal efficiently.

Because it strengthens the entire musculoskeletal system, exercise also helps younger people to resist injuries from falls and high-impact accidents. A client of mine took dance classes two to three times per week and jogged regularly all through her twenties and thirties. During that time she experienced a couple of major falls and one automobile accident—situations that would have likely resulted in bone breaks or severe muscle pulls had her body not been so tough, flexible, and strong from all the physical activities she was doing.

Benefit 11: Organize the Chaos in Your Life

People who live with high levels of responsibility are often the toughest to convince that taking time out of their already busy schedules for exercise will benefit them. But, in practice, time spent exercising actually will give them *more* time because they will be handling their stress better and feeling more calm and focused.

Fifty-five-year-old Donna has a very busy practice as a health care attorney. But five years ago, she herself was not very healthy. "I was working fifty or sixty hours a week, just rushing from one thing to another. I finally went to the doctor because I was having chest pains. They decided it was esophageal spasms probably caused by the chaos in my life, running around and not eating well. It scared me because they did a workup to rule out heart problems. That was negative, but it brought me back to reality. All of a sudden I knew I needed to get some of this stress under control."

After a year of exercising off and on with variable success, Donna decided to try my Pro Circuit Exercise Program. She received an initial health evaluation, met with my nutritionist, and began to work out religiously with my trainer, at least three times a week for an hour and fifteen minutes. Donna balanced out her schedule by leaving work early on the days she trained and going to work earlier on other days.

> I was very de-conditioned when I started, but after a year and a half I had lost thirty pounds and a lot of inches. But it wasn't so much the weight. It's mostly the healthy feeling. The control over not just your body, but also your schedule. It helps organize your life so that a certain portion of your time is going to be focused on you. I observed in my own family, both men and women, but particularly women, become frail—they're just not strong enough to lift things or do things or they have bone breaks. I didn't want to get into that position, I really wanted to feel stronger. I didn't have a lot of upper body strength, but now I do. I don't feel like I live that chaotic lifestyle anymore, even though I am busy at times. You can be busy, if you are balanced and have the energy to do so. When I started, I was worn out. But doing this program is like investing so that you are building up your savings account. If you have a hard day or a hard week, you have the energy to take care of it.

For people of all ages, proper exercise, especially when coupled with wise nutrition, is like an insurance policy helping to keep you healthy and buffering the effects of life's daily stresses.

12

Attain the Maximum Rewards from Exercise

There are three basic components to exercise: frequency, intensity, and time. One way to remember these is to think of the word "FIT."

1. Frequency—exercising frequently enough for you to achieve cumulative results
2. Intensity—exercising within your optimum pro-formance zone
3. Time—the actual length of your exercise session, not counting time in the gym spent getting dressed or socializing

Before starting the Pro Circuit Exercise Program it is important to become familiar with the basic requirements within each of these areas because only then will you get the maximum benefit from your workout.

Intensity: Reach Your Target Training Zone

In order to maximize your Pro Circuit training benefits, you will want to exercise with enough intensity to reach your target training zone. This is the optimum workout heart rate range according to your age and fitness level. A standard formula for finding your target heart rate is 220 minus your age for men and 230 minus your age for women. This figure represents your maximum age-predicted attainable heart rate. You should *never* exceed this heart rate.

- For beginners, 60 percent of maximum is the target training heart rate.
- For relatively fit people, the target is 70 percent of maximum.
- For well-conditioned people and athletes, the target is 80 percent of maximum.

For example, a relatively fit forty-five-year-old man would want to reach and maintain a target heart rate of 123 beats per minute, give or take a few beats ($220 - 45 \times .70 = 123$). A relatively fit forty-five-year-old woman would have a target heart rate of approximately 130 beats per minute ($230 - 45 \times .70 = 130$).

You may also choose to take the gold standard of tests for identifying your target training heart rate known as the pulmonary stress test, which refers to the measurement of the amount of oxygen versus CO_2 you expend while exerting yourself. This test can be administered by either an exercise physiologist or preferably a cardiologist trained in exercise testing. It will provide you with the definitive measurement of your maximum endurance capacity and help you to determine the anaerobic threshold for your training intensity based on your workout objectives.

Monitoring Your Target Heart Rate

Since your goal is to stay within your target heart rate during your entire Pro Circuit workout, you will want to monitor it off and on. One way is to place your finger lightly on your carotid artery, located in your neck, midway between your chin and the hinge of your jaw. You should feel a strong pulse with your finger. Count every beat within a ten-second interval, then multiply by six.

You may also choose to purchase a pulse rate monitor, which you can wear on your wrist, giving you a continual status of your heart rate throughout the training session. I personally always wear a pulse rate monitor and encourage the athletes with whom I work to do the same.

If your pulse is much higher than your target training zone, lesson your exercise intensity by either decreasing the amount of weight you are using, doing fewer repetitions, or slowing down a bit. If your pulse rate is lower than your target training zone, you may want to work harder by increasing your weights and moving more briskly. Should you feel any pain or prolonged discomfort, stop exercising immediately and check with your doctor.

After a while you will be able to sense when you are in your training zone by how you feel as your workout progresses. If you are breezing through the circuit without any apparent exertion, you're probably below your target zone.

Using the Mackie Method of Instinctive Intensity Training: IIT

A second way to make sure your heart rate is within your performance training zone is what I call Instinctive Intensity Training or IIT. Research indicates that the standard heart rate formula overpredicts the maximal heart rate zone for twenty- to twenty-nine-year-olds and underpredicts for forty- to fifty-nine-year-olds. It is also true that a number of medications can affect actual heart rate, such as drugs for lowering blood pressure.

With these caveats in mind, I would like to show you how to monitor your intensity level while doing the Pro Circuit or any other type of exercise using the IIT method.

Everyone has heard the expression "give it a 100 percent effort." But I have learned working with myself and with my individual athletes that you can only give 100 percent for a very short time without becoming totally exhausted and compromising your skill. In reality, the strongest effort that you can maintain consistently is closer to 80 percent of your maximum effort. Therefore, my rule for your training sessions is as follows. After your doctor has cleared you of all exercise restrictions, go to your gym, warm up carefully, then see what you would consider your maximum effort. Once you've identified how that feels, use the following scale to find the appropriate IIT zone for your workout.

THE INSTINCTIVE INTENSITY TRAINING SCALE

IIT Level	Percent of Maximum Effort	Perception
4	40	warm-up effort
6	60	mild effort
7	70	moderate effort
8	80	strong effort
9	90	very strong effort
10	100	maximum effort

The concept behind the IIT Scale is that no one can tell you exactly how many pounds to use or how vigorously you need to exercise. What is easy for one person might be strenuous for another, especially if you are deconditioned, overweight, or haven't exercised for a while. Perceptions will be different for different people.

The goal of finding your appropriate IIT level is to learn to listen to your body. This means paying attention to a broad spectrum of physical sensations, including fatigue levels, muscle or leg pain, physical stress, and shortness of breath. For every activity, you can estimate how hard you feel you are working. Research has shown that your perception of the amount of effort you feel you are putting into an activity is likely to agree with the actual physical measurements of that physical effort. In other words, if your body tells you that you are exercising moderately, measurements of things such as how fast your heart is beating would probably show that it really is working at a moderate level. During moderate activity you can sense that you are challenging yourself but are not yet near your limit.

While doing the Pro Circuit, your goal should be to try to work at level 7 to 8 on the IIT Scale, between "moderate" and "strong." In other words, you should feel that you are making an effort, but it will not be overwhelming or debilitating. As your body adapts and you become more fit, you can gradually add more weight, increase your repetitions, increase your time from thirty minutes to forty-five minutes, and move from one to two or three complete circuits of the series.

One of the advantages of the IIT Scale is that the rate of instinctive or perceived exertion will be the same for everyone, regardless of their age, gender, or actual heart rate (if, for example, you are taking medication that affects your heartbeats per minute).

Frequency and Time: How Often and How Long You Exercise

Since three out of four North Americans are totally or mostly sedentary, almost any level of exercise done ten to twenty minutes a day can have a beneficial effect on the way you feel. This includes even ordinary activities such as walking, taking the stairs instead of the elevator, housecleaning, riding the stationary bike for twenty minutes while watching television or reading the newspaper, gardening, washing the car, and so forth.

To achieve appreciable results, however, studies have shown that you should do aerobic exercises at least three times a week for at least thirty minutes, and resistance exercises two or three times a week, with a day off in between. The reason you need that day off is to give your muscle tissue a chance to repair itself. Many people think that resistance exercises build muscle. This is not true. Resistance exercises tear down muscle tissue. It is the time you take off in between and the nutritious foods you eat that repair your muscles, making them stronger and larger than before. You can, however, do thirty to forty-five minutes of aerobic exercises such as walking or jogging every day of the week without harm, since these exercises don't tear down muscle tissue but build up aerobic capacity.

For maximum results, your goal is to increase your Pro Circuit workout to forty-five minutes. If you have the extra time and develop the aerobic stamina and strength, you may even wish to do the circuit for an hour. Just always stay within your target heart rate zone or your RPE. You will begin to feel your energy, cardiovascular levels, and strength increase after only a month on the program, but you will see maximum results in weight loss, strength gains, and health benefits such as lowered triglycerides and cholesterol within twelve weeks.

In the twelve-week Pro Circuit pilot study done on the New Orleans Police Department, the officers saw an average of a 9 percent increase in HDL (good cholesterol) and a 53 percent decrease in triglycerides. And these officers weren't even on my prescribed nutritional program. We just gave them certain basic nutritional guidelines and instructed them to make sure that they had a shake of 20 grams of Personal Edge soy protein powder in juice or water twice a day, since soy has been shown to reduce cholesterol when taken in conjunction with a low-fat diet. We encouraged them to drink their soy protein shake or to eat a piece of fruit before each workout, since exercising on an empty stomach makes some people feel light-headed.

Consult with Your Doctor Before You Begin

Before beginning any exercise program, it is important that you consult with your doctor, especially if you have not exercised in a while and know or suspect that you have significant health problems. If you have taken the self-evaluation health tests in chapter 8, by now you should have a fairly good idea of the state of your general health.

Another important screening tool is the Physical Activity Readiness Questionnaire, more commonly known as the PAR-Q, included below. This basic self-evaluation, developed by the Canadian Society for Exercise Physiology, has been clinically tested and shown to be an effective and reliable screening tool.

PAR-Q and You
(A Questionnaire for People Ages 15 to 69)

Regular physical activity is fun and healthy, and increasingly more people are starting to become more active every day. Being more active is very safe for most people. However, some people should check with their doctor before they start becoming much more physically active.

If you are planning to become much more physically active than you are now, start by answering the seven questions below. If you are between the ages of fifteen and sixty-nine, the PAR-Q will tell you if you should check with your doctor before you start. If you are over sixty-nine years of age, and you are not used to being very active, check with your doctor.

Common sense is your best guide when you answer these questions. Please read the questions carefully and answer each one honestly, yes or no.

	Yes	No
1. Has your doctor ever said that you have a heart condition *and* that you should only do physical activity recommended by a doctor?	☐	☐
2. Do you feel pain in your chest when you do physical activity?	☐	☐
3. In the past month, have you had chest pain when you were not doing physical activity?	☐	☐
4. Do you lose your balance because of dizziness or do you ever lose consciousness?	☐	☐
5. Do you have a bone or joint problem that could be made worse by a change in your physical activity?	☐	☐
6. Is your doctor currently prescribing drugs (for example, water pills) for your blood pressure or heart condition?	☐	☐
7. Do you know of any *other reason* why you should not do physical activity?	☐	☐

If you answered "Yes" to one or more questions, talk with your doctor by phone or in person before you start becoming more physically active or before you have a fitness appraisal. Tell your doctor about the PAR-Q and which questions you answered "Yes."

- You may be able to do any activity you want—as long as you start slowly and build up gradually. Or you may need to restrict your activities to those that are safe for you. Talk with your doctor about the kinds of activities in which you wish to participate and follow his/her advice.
- Find out which community programs are safe and helpful for you.

If you honestly answered "No" to all *PAR-Q questions,* you can be reasonably sure that you can:

- Start becoming much more physically active—begin slowly and build up gradually. This is the safest and easiest way to go.
- Take part in a fitness appraisal—this is an excellent way to determine your basic fitness so that you can plan the best way for you to live actively.

Delay becoming much more active:

- If you are not feeling well because of a temporary illness such as a cold or a fever—wait until you feel better.
- If you are or may be pregnant—talk to your doctor before you start becoming more active.

Please note: If your health changes so that you then answer "Yes" to any of the above questions, tell your fitness or health professional. Ask whether you should change your physical activity plan.

Informed use of the PAR-Q: The Canadian Society for Exercise Physiology, Health Canada, and their agents assume no liability for persons who undertake physical activity. If in doubt after completing the questionnaire, consult your doctor prior to physical activity.

Now that you have learned the basics about exercising safely and getting the most from your exercise regimen, let's move on to the Pro Circuit Exercise Program.

13

The Pro Circuit Exercise Program

One of the most effective tools I have found to keep the business athlete at the top of his or her form is consistent and correct exercise, especially if combined with proper nutrition and stress management techniques. Beginning and maintaining an exercise program can be very difficult for the man or woman on the fast track who has very little time. That is why I have developed the Pro Circuit, a workout that combines both strength and core training with cardiovascular conditioning.

The beauty of this program is that you can start it at any age and at any level of fitness and make it as challenging as you want. The Pro Circuit is designed to give you maximum benefits for a minimum time investment—thirty to forty-five minutes, three times a week—in as few as eight to twelve weeks. Where you go from there is up to you. The sky is, literally, the limit. I have seen clients in this program lose body fat, gain lean muscle, trim their waistlines, increase their energy levels, improve their health, and learn how to manage their stress successfully. Furthermore, this program is so user-friendly that you will want to make it a permanent part of your routine. You can use any type of selectorized equipment at home or on the road. It's the Pro Circuit philosophy that counts.

Creating the Program

I put the finishing touches on the Pro Circuit Exercise Program when I offered it as a pilot program for the New Orleans Police Department. I noticed right away that the workout programs used by most police officers, both male and female, did not match up to their job descriptions. Most of the officers were heavily involved in strength training, and quite a few in power lifting. Overall, when we tested them, they were overweight, had a high percentage of body fat, and significantly elevated cholesterol and triglyceride levels.

Since police officers spend their time alternating between sitting in the squad car or behind a desk and then engaging in great bursts of activity when they are called to a crime scene, I could see that they needed a workout program that had a significant aerobic component to provide recovery between events. They were moving from machine to machine in the gym, but they weren't elevating their heart rates over a long enough period of time to ensure aerobic fitness. So they lacked physical endurance, which was often necessary in successfully chasing criminals and physically overcoming and arresting them once they were caught. One forty-one-year-old police officer told me that his greatest fear was having his weapon taken from him by a younger criminal during a struggle following a long chase. He knew that, as a rule, younger criminals were faster, leaner, and less winded than he was at the end of a long pursuit.

I had the officers do the Pro Circuit for thirty minutes a day, three times a week, for twelve weeks—giving them general nutritional guidelines. All of the men and women in the program reported weight loss, much greater energy, an increase in lean muscle percentage, drops in cholesterol and triglycerides, more confidence in their ability to successfully manage the physically challenging components of their jobs, and noticeable reduction in levels of stress.

Lieutenant Eddie Selby: Amazed by His Fitness Improvements

Since fifty-one-year-old Lieutenant Eddie Selby began doing the Pro Circuit his weight has remained at 175, but his body fat has dropped to an amazing 7 percent. His waistline is thirty-three inches, his stress level has decreased, and his performance on the job has greatly improved. What Lieutenant Selby appreciates most about the program is the level of aerobic conditioning he's been able to achieve. Like many police officers, he used to concentrate exclusively on strength training. That made him strong, but it did little for his endurance. "We deal with criminals on the street that are constantly running from us. Or they decide that they want to get into a fight with us. If you're in good cardiovascular condition, you're going to be able to outlast them."

Lieutenant Selby is impressed not only with the results he has achieved on the Pro Circuit, but also with the results he has seen in his fellow officers. "One guy lost a hundred pounds. Everybody's triglycerides dropped down. Their body fat dropped, and they started changing from fat to muscle. All of a sudden your clothes start fitting better and you look and feel better. I love clothes and I love dressing well. I know that people form their first opinion of you based on what they see."

With the Pro Circuit Lieutenant Selby doesn't find it difficult to maintain high energy levels, cardiovascular health, and a lean appearance. "The program is very simple. It works wonders."

The Pro Circuit: A Program for Busy Professionals

I designed the Pro Circuit Exercise Program to provide a workout for busy professionals who may not have more than thirty to forty-five minutes to work out in the gym. When time is short, people often have to choose between the two exercise modes—aerobic (exercises such as jogging, walking, riding a stationary bike, or step classes) and resistance (strength training with free weights or machines). If they choose to do primarily aerobic training, their overall cardiovascular fitness can increase by as much as 30 percent and their weight loss will be enhanced, but they will not experience a significant increase in strength and muscle mass. If they choose to spend their limited time doing primarily resistance training, their cardio fitness will not significantly increase, and they will likely lose only about a quarter pound of scale weight per week, even though they will get stronger.

Combine Two Superior Workouts in One

With the Pro Circuit Exercise Program, you no longer have to choose between one mode of exercise or the other because this program is two superior workouts in one. You will be building your cardiovascular (endurance) capacity while substantially increasing your muscle strength *and* increasing your overall flexibility. The Pro Circuit will lower your resting heart rate, reduce your blood pressure, increase your metabolism, and substantially reduce abdominal body fat.

You do not need any special equipment to do the Pro Circuit. You only need a gym or a fitness center that provides selectorized weight training stations (machines where you can adjust the weight by placing a pin in the appropriate slot). Ideally, you should have between ten and fourteen machines that will allow you to alternate between your upper torso, the core area (abdominals, lower back, and hips), lower body, and aerobic stations such as a jogging platform, a stationary bike, a treadmill, or a jump rope.

You will be working for just thirty seconds on each machine, performing twelve to twenty repetitions of an exercise, alternating between upper body, the core area, and lower body. To start, I suggest twelve repetitions for the upper body, twenty for the midbody, and fifteen for the lower body, but you may increase your reps as your fitness level increases. In between each of these exercises you will do some kind of aerobic activity. For example, you might do twelve repetitions of a chest press, take five or ten seconds to move to a stationary bike or pick up a jump rope, then pump or jump vigorously for thirty seconds. Then you will take another five to ten seconds to move on to an abdominal machine, from there to an aerobic station, from there to a leg press, and so on until you have completed a full circuit of ten to fourteen machines.

Achieve peripheral heart conditioning. Alternating between the upper body and the lower body gives you peripheral heart conditioning because you are constantly forcing the blood between these two areas, which improves circulation. By working different parts of the body and resting others, you also avoid the buildup of fatigue and lactic acid in any particular muscle group. While one part of the body is working, the other parts are resting.

How long does a circuit take? Depending on the number of exercises in the circuit, for the average person, each complete Pro Circuit will take about eleven to seventeen minutes, including the ten seconds of transition time between machines. As your conditioning improves, you can gradually add exercise stations and/or complete circuits until you reach your desired fitness level. For best results, you'll want to perform this workout three days a week for thirty to forty-five minutes, with one day off of rest in between. On your days off you can engage in at least thirty minutes of cardiovascular training, such as bicycling, walking, or running if you wish. Forty-five minutes within your appropriate heart rate zone would be preferable if you are carrying extra abdominal fat.

What Results Can You Expect?

A program very similar to the Pro Circuit was tested at the Institute for Aerobics Research in Dallas, Texas, on a group of men and women who were rated as being in average physical condition when they began the study. These individuals worked out for approximately thirty minutes, three days a week for twelve weeks. They achieved dramatic gains in aerobic capacity and strength and substantial reduction in body fat:

- People experienced *significant improvement in their aerobic capacity, 17 percent in the men and 17 percent in the women.* This 15 to 25 percent increase was similar to that reported from running-only programs without the negative impact to knees and ankles. And running doesn't provide the bonus benefit of increased strength and flexibility.
- Both men and women *achieved a 17 percent increase in upper body strength. The men achieved a 21 percent increase in lower body strength and the women a 26 percent increase.*
- *The men lost an average of 17 percent body fat and the women lost 11 percent.* Since losing unwanted fat is the goal of most exercise programs, this type of exercise program is ideal for that purpose.

The Pro Circuit: Dramatic Results in a Variety of Settings

I have used the Pro Circuit Exercise Program in a variety of settings with excellent results each time. Let me share with you some stories about the people whom this system has helped.

I began developing the Pro Circuit back in the days when I was preparing Riddick Bowe for a boxing match with Jorge Luis Gonzalez. The sport of boxing requires tremendous physical strength coupled with short periods of great stamina and endurance. Yet at the time the accepted method of coaching boxers was almost exclusively aerobic in nature. This didn't make sense to me because I knew that what boxers did was to release enormous bursts of energy in each round and then to rest in between. A different type of workout was required.

When I had Riddick Bowe doing a form of the Pro Circuit four times a week, we saw dramatic body changes. Bowe ended up being able to perform over 700 repetitions within forty-five minutes and achieved his highest recorded lean body mass (218.94 pounds) and his lowest body fat percentage (9.9 percent). He beat Gonzalez in that fight. We used the same Pro Circuit training concept to enable him to take back his heavyweight title from Evander Holyfield during Bowe versus Holyfield III.

As You Begin the Pro Circuit, Ten Things to Keep in Mind

As you begin your first Pro Circuit workout, there are several guidelines you should keep in mind.

1. *Orient yourself with the equipment.* One of the first things you should do before you begin is to thoroughly familiarize yourself with the selectorized weight training machines that you plan to use in your gym. One of the gym's trainers can show you how to properly position your body for each exercise and can demonstrate proper lifting and breathing techniques. The trainer can also help you to select the proper starting weight for each machine.
2. *Always warm up your muscles first* with five or ten minutes of light calisthenics or stretching exercises involving all parts of your body. Also do a warm-up aerobic exercise such as cycling or jogging in place to bring your pulse rate up toward the lowered end of your target heart rate zone.
3. *Move quickly between stations or machines.* Work at a quick but controlled pace at each station and move briskly between stations. This steady and consistent movement will help to maintain your target heart rate. If you need to, practice adjusting the equipment seat and weights beforehand so that you can easily adjust the machine to your own specifications.

   The time you take to move from station to station should be 15 seconds for beginners, 10 to 15 seconds for intermediates, and 5 to 10 seconds for those who are advanced.

4. *Lift moderate weights.* When you are using a machine, lift only the amount of weight you can comfortably lift 12 to 20 times, depending on the body part you are working, within 30 seconds. The correct amount of weight will be enough to make you feel as if you have reached the point of muscle fatigue by the end of your required reps. If it's too much weight, you won't be able to complete the set. Too little weight and you won't feel muscle tiredness at the end of your reps. Each lifting stroke should be relatively fast, with a well-controlled return. If you are not sure how much weight you should be lifting, ask a trainer. Don't risk injuring yourself.

   While you will attempt to increase your weight slightly each week or so to keep your body changing, never compromise your form, stability, alignment, or posture to increase the number of pounds you are lifting. The result is almost certain to be injury and poor posture. The best way to build strength is to maintain proper position and form during your workout, even if you are using only a relatively light amount of weight. Play it safe and never try to handle more weight than your body can stabilize.

5. *Maintain correct body positioning.* The most efficient position for the body while doing resistance training is one in which the spine is in a neutral position with a slight degree of straightening in the thoracic region (upper chest). This is accomplished by positioning yourself comfortably against the backrest of the machine, then pushing your shoulders back slightly (known as "scapular retraction") and lifting your chest slightly up and out. Positioning the spine in this manner is more efficient for supporting weight while still allowing for the least amount of intervertebral disk compression in the cervical (neck) and lumbar (lower back) regions. Also contract your abdominal muscles during lifting to help stabilize the lumbar spine.

6. *Don't forget to breathe.* Keeping respiration going will keep your blood pressure from rising. Depending on the exercise, inhale when you extend and exhale on the way back in; inhale on the way down and exhale on the way out.

7. *Complete all repetitions for each machine.* If the weight becomes heavy, stop the set, reduce the weight, and continue until you have completed the set of repetitions.

8. *Stay hydrated.* Make sure that you carry a bottle of water with you when exercising and take frequent drinks. You will want to drink between one half and one entire 1.5-liter bottle of water per hour of workout time.

9. *Always cool down.* Finish your workout with a cooldown to decrease your pulse and breathing rates. Gradually reduce the intensity level until your pulse returns to a normal resting state. Then perform some easy, static stretching exercises using the stretch strap routine or other stretching exercises you enjoy doing to loosen tight muscles and increase flexibility.

10. *Build up your routine.* If thirty minutes seems too challenging to begin with, start your Pro Circuit conservatively by trying to complete one fifteen-minute circuit per day, three days per week. Gradually work up to two fifteen-minute circuits per session three times a week.

   At this point you'll begin to see some definite results in both your aerobic and muscular fitness.

A Sample Pro Circuit Workout

The following are pictures of fourteen exercises with correct positioning and a description of how to do each one correctly. This is just a sample program. Any group of resistance and aerobic exercises done to the specifications described previously is acceptable.

I have also included a sample progress chart for you at the end of the exercise sequence.

CHEST PRESS

1. Sit on the bench with your feet flat on the floor and slightly wider than shoulder width apart.
2. Grasp the handles and push outward until your arms are extended.
3. Return to the starting position and repeat for the required reps.

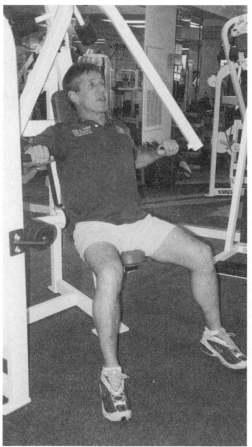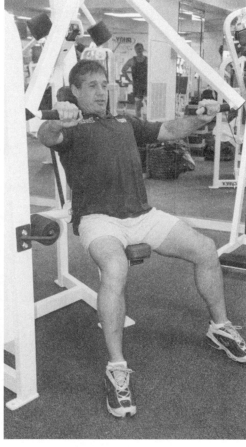

CALF RAISE

1. Stand on the edge of the platform, knees slightly bent with your heels extending off the platform. The pads should be resting on your shoulders.
2. Rise up on your toes and hold for three to five seconds.
3. Lower your heels to the starting position and repeat for the required reps.

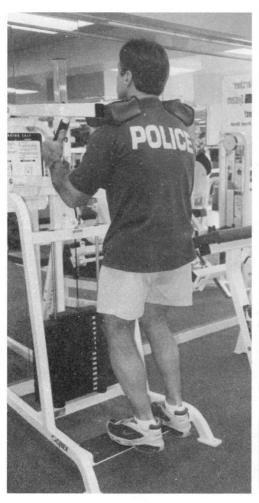
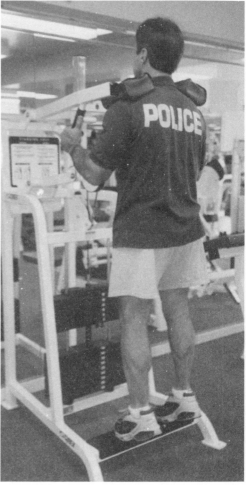

ARM CURL

1. Sit at the machine, your feet flat on the floor and slightly wider than shoulder width apart. Grasp the handles with your palms upward, upper arms resting on the pad.
2. Curl your arms up until they form a 90-degree bend at the elbow.
3. Return to the starting position and repeat for the required reps.

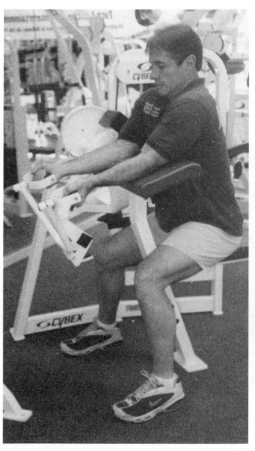
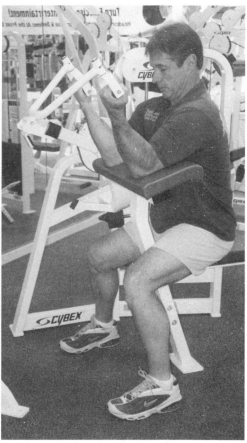

BACK EXTENSION

1. Sit on the bench with your feet solidly on the platform. The pad should be resting just below your shoulders on your upper back.
2. Push back on the pad to extend your back to a prone position. Do not overextend.
3. Return to the starting position and repeat for the required reps.

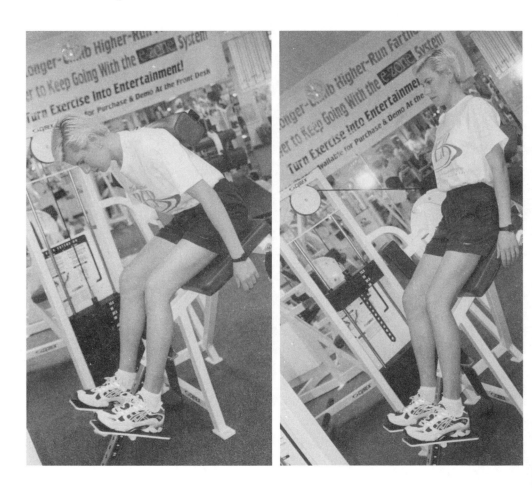

SEATED ROW

1. Sit on the bench, feet flat on the floor and slightly wider than shoulder width apart. Your arms should be extended.
2. Grasp the handles with your palms facing down and pull back on the bars until your arms are bent at a 90-degree angle at the elbow. Do not let your elbows go past this point.
3. Return to the starting position and repeat for the required reps.

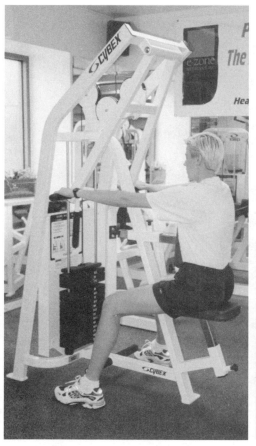
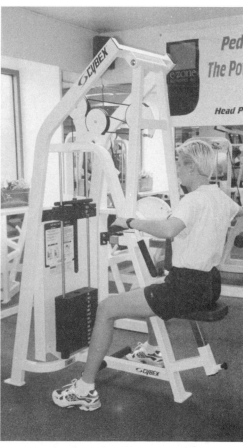

LEG EXTENSION

1. Sit on the bench with your back supported by the pad. Place your legs behind the footpads at the ankles.
2. Raise your legs until they are extended straight out. Do not overextend.
3. Return to the starting position and repeat for the required reps.

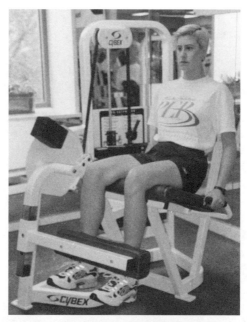

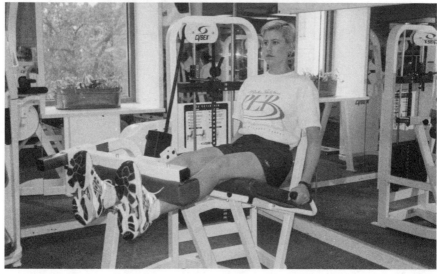

SEATED ROTATION

1. Lie on the bench, hooking your legs under the pads for support. Hold a medicine ball between your hands and slightly above your waist. Contract abdominals during exercise.
2. Rise up into a crunch position and move the ball from side to side for the required reps.
3. Rotate your entire upper torso as you turn.

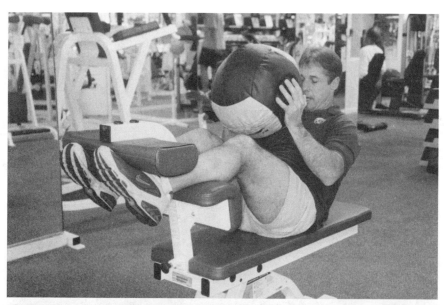

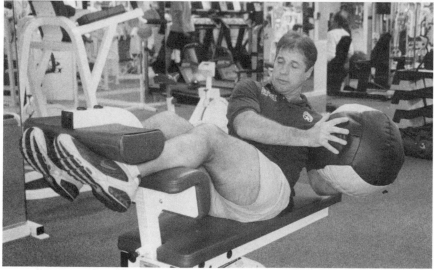

CHEST FLYS

1. Sit on the bench with your feet flat on the floor and slightly wider than shoulder width apart. Place your arms against the pads so that they are parallel to your body. Do not overextend. Your elbows should be slightly lower than your shoulders.
2. Bring the pads together with your elbows still lower than your shoulders.
3. Return to the starting position and repeat for the required reps.

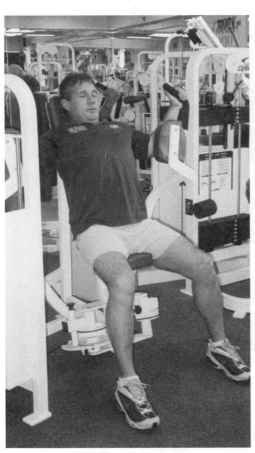 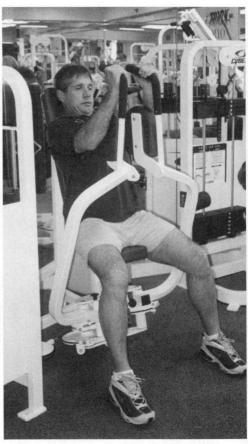

LEG CURL

1. Lie on your stomach on the bench. Grasp the handles provided for support. Place your legs under the bar at the ankle.
2. Curl your legs upward until your knees are at a 90-degree angle. Do not go past 90 degrees.
3. Return to the starting position and repeat for the required reps.

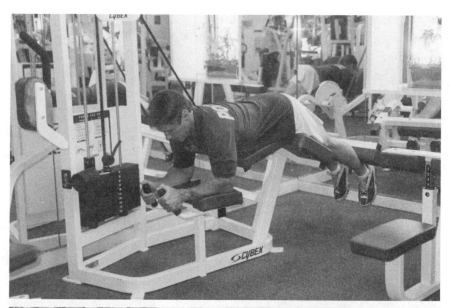

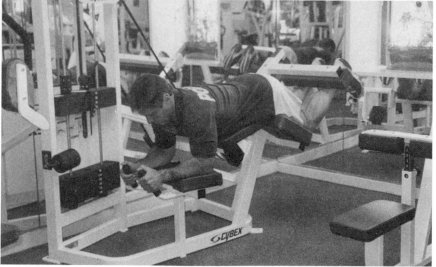

LAT PULLDOWN

1. Sit at the machine with the bar above your thighs for support. Grasp the handles overhead with your palms facing in.
2. Pull down on the handles until they are close to your chest.
3. Return to the starting position and repeat for required reps.

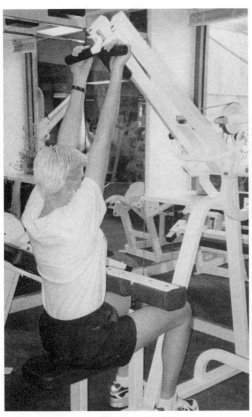
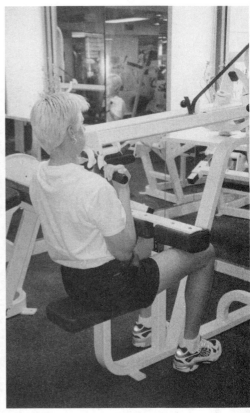

Seated Crunch

1. Sit on the bench with your feet flat on the floor and slightly wider than shoulder width apart. Your arms should be resting on the pad so that they are at a 90-degree angle from your body.
2. Tighten your abdominal muscles and bend forward, pushing the pad downward.
3. Return to the starting position and repeat for the required reps.

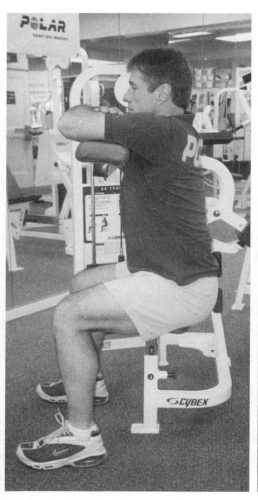
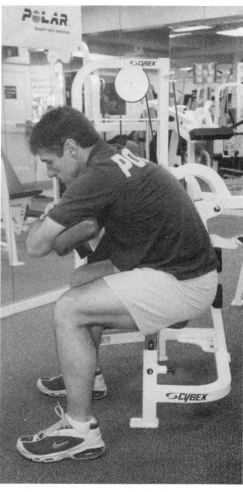

TRICEP PRESS

1. Sit on the bench with your feet flat on the floor and slightly wider than shoulder width apart. Grasp the handles with your palms facing inward, your elbows on the pads and bent at a 90-degree angle.
2. Press the bars down until your arms are extended straight out.
3. Return to the starting position and repeat for the required reps.

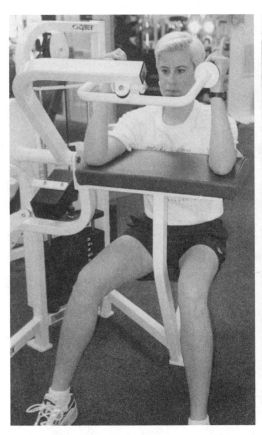
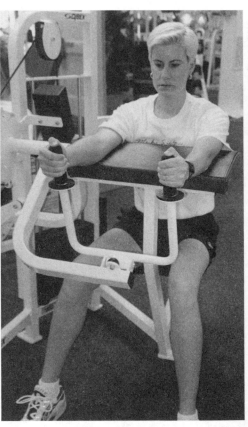

LEG PRESS

1. Sit on the bench so that your knees are at an angle of no more than 90 degrees. Grasp the handles for support.
2. Push on the platform with your feet until your legs are extended, keeping your knees slightly bent. Do not overextend.
3. Return to the starting position and repeat for the required reps.

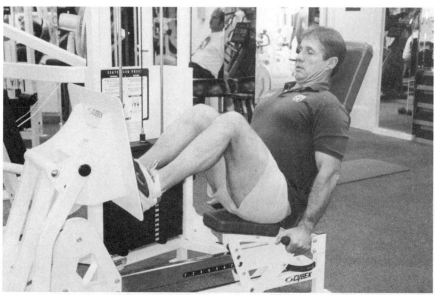

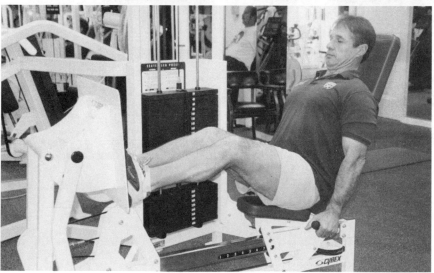

SHOULDER PRESS

1. Sit on the bench with your feet flat on the floor, slightly wider than shoulder width apart. Support your back on the pad provided.
2. Grasp the handles with your palms facing in, then push up on the bars until your arms are extended to a point where your shoulders are level and your elbows are at a 90-degree angle. Do not cause impingement.
3. Return to the starting position and repeat for required reps.

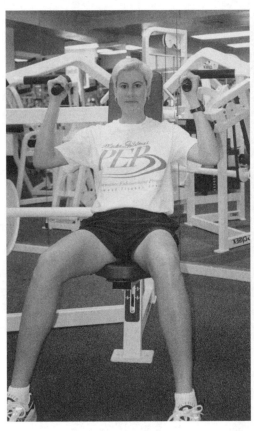 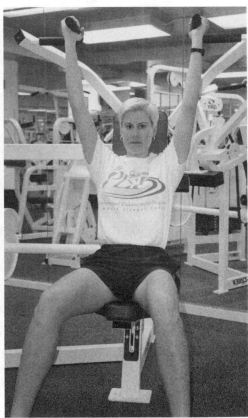

PRO CIRCUIT SEQUENCE AND TRACKING CHART

Start: Weight _____ **Waist** _____ **BMI** _____ **Body Fat %** _____

Target	WEEK											
HR _____	1	2	3	4	5	6	7	8	9	10	11	12
Exercise Order												
Chest Press												
Calf Raise												
Arm Curl												
Back Extension												
Seated Row												
Leg Extension												
Seated Rotation												
Chest Flys												
Leg Curl												
Lat Pulldown												
Seated Crunch												
Tricep Press												
Leg Press												
Shoulder Press												
Repeat after Each Exercise Bike or Jog in Place or Stationary Device												

Week 2   Weight_____   Waist_____   BMI_____   Body Fat %_____

Week 4   Weight_____   Waist_____   BMI_____   Body Fat %_____

Week 6   Weight_____   Waist_____   BMI_____   Body Fat %_____

Week 8   Weight_____   Waist_____   BMI_____   Body Fat %_____

Week 10   Weight_____   Waist_____   BMI_____   Body Fat %_____

Week 12   Weight_____   Waist_____   BMI_____   Body Fat %_____

As Hans Seyle said, all of us have an energy savings account and a checking account. Once the checking account is overdrawn, our body has no choice but to go into its savings account, the very life force. If we draw too much out of that account, we become ill and eventually kill ourselves. But if we make aerobic and strength training a part of our lives, we will never reach that place where we are scraping the bottom. We will be able to live long, healthy, energetic, and deeply fulfilling lives.

PART THREE

Cultivate Your Passion for Your Life and Work

14

Recharge Your Passion for Your Career

Your success in your career will always be in direct proportion to whether or not you can feel a real passion for your work. If I had to choose just one question to ask readers, it would be, "Does your job fill you with passion?"

One of the lessons that professional boxing has taught me is that passion is everything. I have often seen boxers go up against opponents with greater talent, but they were victorious because they had the greatest passion for victory and the greatest love for what they do. There may come a point where your competitor may have more talent than you, but if you can maintain and nurture the fires of your passion, you will be able to endure in your profession long after your opponent is gone. Passion is the pure energy that helps you to survive by constantly growing and reinventing yourself and your life.

When you feel passion about your vocation, you will give off a high level of energy and enthusiasm. Coworkers will have a more positive perception of you. I'm not talking about the kind of hyperactive person who can't sit still, but about someone who makes everyone's energy level rise and the room expand when he starts talking. This person chooses his words with care. He does not say, "I hope we will be on top when the dust clears," but "Without a doubt, with all of our resources and the talent in this room, we're going to be on top when the dust clears." This type of energy, confidence, and determination inspires others to believe that anything is possible.

193

Three Options to Regain Your Passion

There are as many ways to recover your passion for your job as there are people. But during my decades of working with professional athletes and people in all type of business endeavors, I have found that there are three basic options for regaining your passion. If your present job seems flat and unchallenging, you can either:

1. Work to recover your passion for the job you have.
2. Make a lateral move into another area of your profession.
3. Change careers.

Option 1: Work to Recover Your Passion for the Job You Have

Feeling passionate about your work is not a given. It is a quality that you must constantly strive to nurture and maintain. Like any other situation in life, such as marriage, parenting, or your tennis game, keeping your interest in your job alive is an ongoing process. It takes self-awareness and effort.

Evaluate Your Job Satisfaction

Any time you feel that you have lost your passion for your career, it is time to do a self-audit. Stop and take a discerning look at how the job is affecting you, because the workplace is where you spend most of your waking hours. It's important to ask yourself whether you feel happy and fulfilled, whether you still feel challenged, and whether your job is adversely affecting your overall health and well-being. Begin by filling out the simple Job Satisfaction Questionnaire.

Job Satisfaction Questionnaire

1. **Job Satisfaction:** On a scale of 1 to 10, where 1 represents no satisfaction and 10 represents totally satisfied, how would you rate your job? _____ Can you think of three specific changes in your approach to work, in your relationship with your coworkers, or in the workplace itself that would make your satisfaction level rise to 8 or above?

   1. _____

   2. _____

   3. _____

2. **Stress:** On a scale of 1 to 10, where 1 represents no stress and 10 represents extremely stressful, how would you rate yourself on the job stress scale? _____ What three specific changes could you make to lower your stress levels below 3?

   1. _____

   2. _____

   3. _____

3. **Room for growth:** Do you feel that there is room for you to grow in your career, or do you feel stuck? Yes _____ No _____ Name three ways you could grow in your current job.

   1. _____

   2. _____

   3. _____

4. **Your ideal career.** Describe three characteristics of your ideal career.

   1. _____

   2. _____

   3. _____

   Does your current job match your ideal career? Yes _____ No _____ Is there anything you can do to bring your job closer to your ideal career?

   _____

   _____

   _____

5. **Financial satisfaction:** Do you feel satisfied with the amount of money you make? Yes _____ No _____ Does it seem commensurate with the amount of effort you invest in your job? Yes _____ No _____

6. **Time:** Do you feel that you are working too many hours a week in proportion to the rewards you get from your job? Yes _____ No _____

7. **Family and personal life:** Does your job allow you to have a balanced family and personal life? Yes _____ No _____ If not,

name three things you could do to create a better balance between work and personal life.

1. _____

2. _____

3. _____

Four Ways to Restore Passion in Your Current Job

After filling out the questionnaire, some readers may feel that they want to skip ahead to the sections on making a lateral move or changing careers. But if you feel that your satisfaction level for your current job is high, then here are some practical suggestions for regaining your enthusiasm in the workplace.

1. Visualize solutions to work-related problems. Focused visualization exercises are terrific tools for finding solutions for problems at work. I developed one such visualization technique that I have found helpful over my years of practice. Totally relax your body, one part at a time. Deep, even breathing will help you to relax. Once you feel that you are in a totally relaxed and receptive state, picture yourself inside a blue frame. Now bring the problem at work into the frame. This might take the form of yourself and a coworker having an argument, you trying to communicate with your boss, or a meeting room where you and your colleagues are working on a project together.

Step outside the frame and turn around and look back at your essence. What do you see? Do you see a person who looks frustrated, stressed, concerned? Observe the expression on your face. Do you see anger or impatience there? Walk around yourself. What kind of signals are you giving others with your body language? What do the people around you look like? What are they saying? How do you feel when you look at them, listen to them? What sort of emotions are on their faces when they look at you?

Once you have seen all that you can, step back into your body and imagine that your heart and your mind are powerfully linked together. Now, ask yourself: "What is the solution to this problem?" Allow an image to appear. It might be crystal clear or it might be somewhat foggy and indistinct. It could be a metaphor or something literal, such as a picture of yourself being more patient and carefully listening to a coworker. Stay with that image for a while and learn as much as you can about it.

Then, keeping the link between your heart and your brain open, ask yourself what things you need to do in your life to achieve that solution. Don't try to *make* something happen. Just have faith that your own internal wisdom will bring forth an answer. Know that your subconscious mind is speaking to you, giving you information to which you normally would not have access. Be patient. If this doesn't work the first time, know that you can come back and keep trying. Also know that you can always return to this image to get more information.

Slowly allow yourself to come out of the visualization, then sit for a while with a notebook and write down what you saw and felt. Again, don't try to impose your will on the "solution." Just let the energy flow.

2. Plug energy leaks. Do the people with whom you work give you energy or do they take energy from you in an unhealthy way? It's hard to maintain your passion when you are constantly trying to cope with someone who is a downer. Sometimes you need to put a healthy distance physically—or at least mentally—between yourself and someone at the office who is constantly draining your energy. Don't allow yourself to become enmeshed with a coworker who drains your energy.

Another major energy drain is spending time worrying about things in the office over which you have no control. Intelligent and balanced concern for the things you *do* have some control over is one thing, but worry diminishes your ability to see situations clearly and to get perspective on your job.

Nothing kills passion like energy-draining anxiety and worry. To nurture your passion and keep your energy levels high, I suggest the following:

- Identify unnecessary worries. Practice the internal discipline of not allowing the mind to ruminate about them.
- If you trust in some kind of higher power, give your worries over to that power.
- Don't keep your worries to yourself. Do something about them. Talk your worries out with a trusted friend, family member, or counselor.

3. Capitalize on the strengths of your team. One way to keep your passion alive is to realize that you are not an island unto yourself. We are all members of groups, of teams, of networks of people. Many people lose their passion for their work because they spread themselves too thin and fall apart, thinking they can do everything.

If passion is energy, you need to be able to satisfy and fulfill your passion without burning yourself out. That sometimes means learning how to inspire the team with which you work or the people whom you employ in your organization. I have adopted this principle with my staff at the Mackie Shilstone Center for Performance Enhancement and Lifestyle Management. I have made sure to acknowledge and capitalize on the talented people whom I have mentioned by giving them their own special niches in my program. Chris Depolo is someone who has studied with me to become an expert on sports-specific training, and I have made him my expert on high school programs. I created the Nate Singleton Strength and Speed Camp within my program so that Nate's talents could be showcased. I have done all I can to acknowledge the exceptional work of my nutritionist Molly Kimball by positioning her prominently in my first book, *Lose Your Love Handles.*

If you expect to keep your own passion alive, then you have a responsibility to keep alive the passion of the people who work with you or for you by giving them their own identity. A person whose talents are acknowledged knows where he or she stands within the team. He or she will tend to be more loyal, more creative, and more committed. When a victory is won, spread the credit around. You create a successful team when every individual feels a sense of accomplishment.

4. Prioritize. If you feel exhausted, unfocused, and never seem to have enough hours in the day to get things done, it becomes hard to feel any passion or enthusiasm for your job. At this point, it is time to sit down with a pencil and a piece of paper and begin prioritizing work activities, family, friendships, and social obligations. Ask yourself honestly whether or not you really have to do all of these things or whether you are being driven by guilt or an unbalanced sense of your own importance.

A friend of mine named Susan has a husband, daughter, parents who are in poor health, and a challenging job as a systems designer at a major pharmaceutical company. In spite of all these commitments, Susan felt obligated to do an enormous amount of volunteer work. She was a deacon for her church, ran the local cancer drive, was president of her neighborhood pool, vice president of her women's club, and star of their yearly fund-raiser for Children's Hospital. She was getting four hours sleep a night and catching every cold and flu that came to town.

When Susan came to me for a health and fitness evaluation, she shared with me how overwhelmed she felt. When I suggested that she sit down and prioritize her life, Susan got a clear picture of how unbalanced her life had become. She dropped most of her volunteer work, focused more time on her job and her family, and asked her siblings to take turns driving her elderly parents to their doctors' appointments. Once she was getting enough sleep, eating right, and finding some time to exercise, she rediscovered her old love and passion for the job she does so well. Since then Susan has been promoted to project leader, a job that fully utilizes her excellent people skills and organizational abilities.

Option 2: Make a Lateral Move

Sometimes your passion for your job will begin to wane because you yourself are growing and changing. *Nothing in life remains the same.* The job that once filled you with passion might no longer satisfy you because you are a different person than when you first took the position. Perhaps you are experiencing burnout or no longer feeling challenged. Or maybe changes within the organization for which you work have made the nature of your job less rewarding, pleasurable, or interesting.

At such times you need to sit down with a piece of paper or a trusted friend or mentor and conduct a self-audit. If you find that you still love the type of work you do, but have lost passion for your particular job, then it might be time to make a lateral move into another type of job in your field.

When making a lateral move, it is important to be clear about what your strengths, special talents, and core values about life are. Dean's story below beautifully illustrates these points.

Dean's Story: A Career Move Should Parallel Your Core Values

Dean is thirty-seven years old and currently runs the Evergreen Wellness Center. Although Dean has found the type of work that most completely engages his passion, he had to make two lateral moves in the field of psychotherapy and counseling in order to finally find his most fulfilling niche.

Dean began his adult life studying to be a priest, but as he got closer to his ordination, he realized that what he really wanted to do was to move into the counseling field. His first job was working at a psychiatric hospital with patients on the sexual trauma and addictive disorder units. For four years he worked on the front lines of some very serious mental health issues. Although this work was emotionally demanding, Dean felt fulfilled and challenged because he was learning some very valuable therapy skills. He achieved a high degree of success helping emotionally damaged clients who had strong defense mechanisms.

After a few years, however, Dean began to burn out at this job. One of Dean's core values had always been that he wanted to be an instrument of healing. However, the constant strain he was experiencing in his work was taking its toll on him. "Dealing with individuals who had been so severely emotionally wounded took a lot of energy out of me because I had to provide a safe container for them. At the end of the day, I often felt a strong emotional drain. I had a sense that I couldn't do that too much longer."

In the end, what finally pushed him into making a lateral career move was the disheartening amount of downsizing that was going on in the mental health industry at that time. "The ratio of care providers was decreasing, and the cost to the client was increasing. This was a setup for professional burnout. It lead me to a crossroads where I needed to make a move or my body was going to make that move for me. I was either going to get physically sick or I was going to bottom out."

Dean began to experience high levels of stress. Even though he was exhausted all the time, he wasn't sleeping well. And as the demands of his job got stronger, the activities he usually engaged in to rest his body and revive his spirits began to go by the wayside. He simply no longer had the energy to exercise regularly or to fix a decent meal instead of picking up fast food on the way home. His relationships with family and friends were suffering as well. His wife, who also worked hard, was beginning to feel the strain of his lack of emotional availability.

Even though he was doing work that he loved, Dean began to realize that he needed to do it in another environment, one that would allow him enough downtime to take care of his body and soul.

The solution for him was gradually to begin making the transition into private practice. He did this in stages, continuing part time at the hospital to maintain a financial base while gradually building a practice. This allowed him to set up the parameters of his work in such a way that he could reclaim his life.

Dean strongly feels that any transition we make in our chosen field will only succeed if it reflects the core values in our lives that feed our souls. If what we are doing matches these values, then we will feel fulfilled. If not, then we begin to dry up creatively or become burned out. He also emphasizes that even if we have the "right" job, not having an overall balance in our lives will lead to internal disharmony. "At the hospital, I was engaged in the service that I knew I loved, but the situation didn't allow me time to recharge my batteries."

Currently, Dean is in the process of making a third career shift into what he calls life coaching work. "There is always some kind of parallel process that goes on between our lives and our work. When I was dealing with the high intensity emotions of my clients at the psychiatric hospital, I was also in a phase of life where I needed to attend to a lot of charged emotions in my own life. In the field of psychotherapy, however, the natural step following the healing of emotional pain is learning how to connect with the soul and empower the true self." Life coaching is about taking the elements of the client's present life that he or she wishes to enhance and coaching them about how to do that as quickly as possible. Dean sees his work as empowering people to create the life that they really want to live.

Lateral Move Questionnaire

Below are eight questions to help you determine if you should make a lateral move in your field.

	Yes	No
1. I love the kind of work I do, but not my current job description.	☐	☐
2. I feel that my talents and qualifications are being fully utilized.	☐	☐
3. I feel as if there is room for growth in my job.	☐	☐
4. My boss and my coworkers challenge me in positive ways.	☐	☐
5. I enjoy this kind of work, but some mornings I wake up asking myself, Is this all there is? Is this all I'll ever be?	☐	☐

	Yes	No

6. Recent reorganization has made it difficult for me   ☐   ☐
    to do my job in the way I wish to do it.
7. When I first came to work here, this job was aligned   ☐   ☐
    with my core life values. Now things have changed.
8. I have outgrown this job and am ready for greater   ☐   ☐
    challenges.

Option 3: Change Your Career

Sometimes, no matter what you do, you cannot recapture the passion you once had for your work. Perhaps as you've filled out the self-evaluation questionnaires in this chapter, it's become clear to you that you no longer feel passion for your job and wish to make a career change.

People employ different personal styles and strategies when making a career change. Some prefer to have everything completely figured out before they make their next move. They want to already have their next job lined up before they quit their present job. Others require downtime in which to self-evaluate and explore possibilities. Whichever style best fits you is the one that you will be most comfortable about. The following suggestions may be of use to you, as well as my own story about how I made a change in my own career.

Take Some Time Off to Evaluate Your Options

If you are overwhelmed by the daily grind, it can be difficult to find the time to become clear about your next career move. If you decide that you need to take some time off to find clarity and reassess your skills and career options, find out if you can afford to do that. Sit down with your financial planner and find out what sorts of assets you actually have. Take a realistic look at how much money is coming in, how much is going out, and how it is being spent. You may be surprised to see that you spend much more than you actually need to.

If you decide to take time off for reassessment, make good use of that time. Actively explore new job possibilities, even if that means going back to school or working with a mentor to help you make the change.

I know a man, Ted, who runs the most successful prison aftercare program in the country. Ted used to be a highly successful doctor but felt that his life lacked meaning and challenge. He took stock of his financial assets, decided to sell his practice, and went back to the university to earn a doctoral degree in education and social work. Even though his job of running the prison aftercare program and finding funding sources for it is not easy, the rewards more than make up for the challenges. The deep satisfaction that Ted feels when he sees how 90 percent of the former offenders who graduate from his program turn their lives around and become good parents and hardworking, tax-paying citizens, makes his life worthwhile. He wanted a new career where he felt that he could make a fundamental difference, and he found it.

My Own Story: Seeking Out a Mentor to Help Me Identify My Passion

One of the best ways to find out what kind of work can best feed your passion is to seek the help of a trusted friend and/or mentor, someone who knows you well, and ask him to give you an honest evaluation of your talents. None of us can ever see ourselves as others do, and we often have blind spots to special qualities in our nature.

I myself faced this kind of situation a few years back when I took stock of my life and realized that I had done and achieved so much that nothing lit a fire in me anymore. I really wasn't sure if I wanted to continue with the type of work I do. I was facing some really tough challenges, and I was concerned with where I was going next. I even began to ask my financial adviser if it would be possible for me to retire at age fifty-two.

Everything changed for me, however, when I sought advice from my good friend Steve Wynn, a man of tremendous vision for whom I have the utmost respect. Steve immediately perceived my longing for a change in my life. He didn't tell me that I would be crazy to walk away from my success. Instead, he encouraged me to go out and try new things. "You need to look at something, think about it, and try it first before you make that move. And at your age and at your level of talent and expertise, it's going to be a bold move. If the desire to do something is in your gut and the fire is there, your success will be guaranteed." He also shared his own experience of refocusing and how that had enriched and increased *his* level of passion. I could hear the energy in his voice and feel it in his every movement. And I felt inspired and fired by it.

Before I talked to Steve, I was just going through the motions of my work. I'd been working at my job for twenty-five years, but I had lost much of my enthusiasm. Steve helped me to remember my calling. He reminded me what it had taken for me to achieve the kind of reputation that made top-notch professionals such as Steve Wynn and thousands of outstanding athletes want to work with me in the first place. He rekindled my passion to be the best in the world at performance enhancement and lifestyle management.

This passion gave me the energy to begin focusing on many targets at one time. I decided to create a new company, Mackie Shilstone Incorporated, so that I could establish alternate revenue sources. I also made a commitment to begin sharing my knowledge about fitness and health with readers in the form of books that could reach a larger audience than I could on my own. My newfound passion enabled me to promote my last book, *Lose Your Love Handles,* with so much energy and focus that it went into its third printing three and a half weeks after publication. Less than a year later it had reached its seventh printing.

If you feel your passion slipping and think that it's time for your next move, seek out a trusted adviser to help you invoice your qualities and talents. Sit down and make a list of the things in life that really matter to you, that really make you feel excited. Go out and try new things, even if it means making a bold move, such as starting up your own company, changing careers, or even relocating to a more favorable part of the country. Without passion, life loses its meaning. Don't settle for second best. You owe it to yourself and your family to create a life that truly represents who you are and what you have to offer the world.

Finding a New Passion at Retirement

It is never too late to invest in a new career that you feel passionate about. While some people see retirement as a time to sit in the sun or play golf, more and more men and women today are creating meaningful careers for themselves beyond retirement. This is especially true of the dynamic and entrepreneurial baby boomer generation. After forty years of living an active and productive work life, they are not willing to rest on their laurels.

I remember when a famous quarterback retired from an NFL team at age forty. Soon afterward, he successfully negotiated a new job as a commentator for network sports. He certainly didn't need the money. But he couldn't conceive of living without work for which he felt passion.

One of the main psychological adjustments for anyone in a similar position is that you are now in a position where you find yourself saying, "I remember when I did that." This is a hard statement for anyone to make after they have retired. It makes them feel less important and diminishes their passion because they feel they are living in the past or trying to bring the past into the less-happy present.

The solution is to change your perspective, realizing instead that you have the expertise to know when someone is making the right play because your lifetime of experience tells you the right way to do it. Then you are living in the present. When you have distinguished yourself in a long and illustrious career, people are aware of what you have accomplished. You no longer have to sell yourself to them. Instead, let your love of your work and the wisdom you possess ignite your passion and enthusiasm as you share your knowledge with others who want to learn from your experience.

For example, the father of a client of mine retired and decided to go into local politics. Elected as a town councilman, he was immediately invited to head up the teams that are undertaking the restoration of the town's historic landmarks and the building of recreational sites such as the new marina. As a highly respected and successful engineer and contractor with decades of experience, he has the knowledge to guide others to make the right decisions, both economically and practically. Even though he is in his sixties, there are few men or women in that town who could do this job as well as he can.

With passion comes energy. With energy comes enthusiasm. With enthusiasm anyone can believe in himself or herself. And with belief, the impossible is possible.

15

Renew Your Motivation

In my twenty-five years as a performance enhancement consultant, I've noticed that many athletes do well in the early part of the game but tend to fall apart in the last quarter. The same is true generally for people in the latter part of their careers.

The first twenty-five years of work life are filled with a sense of forward motion and accomplishment. In the years immediately following college, we focus on applying the skills we've learned, creating a strong résumé, and building a career track. Then for the next twenty years or so we mature in that career, gaining experience. Around the age of fifty, however, many men and women begin to lose their confidence, their edge, and their ability to perform as well as they used to. Yet they still have ten or twenty years to go until retirement. Our cultural expectation is that this is just the way it is: people hit midlife and gradually begin to lose the qualities and abilities that sent them to the top.

A Decline in Performance Is Not Inevitable

While a shift in strengths and tactics does occur as one gets older, a decline in performance and creativity is *not* inevitable as people journey through their fifties and sixties. Entrepreneur Lee Iococca's greatest successes with Chrysler came after the age of fifty. And look at great artists such as the painter Pablo Picasso, musical composer Igor Stravinsky, and choreographer Martha Graham. They all did their best work in the later years of their lives.

A client of mine saw Graham's choreography of the *Rite of Spring* in New York City several years ago. Graham was in her nineties when she created this dance—and it was spectacular. When she had reached her forties, the age at which many dancers retire, the innovative Graham had switched her tactics and began designing highly dramatic and less strenuous roles for herself that enabled her to dance into the seventh decade of her life. She no longer had the stamina of youth, but she had incredible presence and charisma, acting ability, and technique. When she finally quit dancing in her seventies, she continued to be one of the world's most innovative choreographers.

In my experience, there are certain specific factors that cause a slowing down of one's powers—and these factors are both *identifiable* and *controllable.* Just as you do not have to fall apart physically as you age, automatically developing high cholesterol, heart disease, low energy levels, lack of mental clarity, and weight gain, you do not have to resign yourself to mediocre performance in your later years.

Let's take a look at some of the factors that, unchecked, could lead to a loss of performance, and then examine some of the steps and creative solutions you can take to overcome these factors and keep yourself motivated and energetic—eager to get out of bed and face the day.

Five Factors that Lead to a Decline in Career Performance

1. Lack of Focus

Many of us seem to lose our focus as we age, becoming more scattered in the way we approach our jobs. Far too many of us find ourselves feeling as if we have already accomplished all our goals and objectives and do not feel focused or energized enough to begin setting new ones. Depression sets in when there seems to be nothing further to look forward to, leading to further lack of energy and ability to concentrate.

The emotional and physiological changes that occur in midlife contribute to our loss of focus. For many of us, midlife is the time when our children are leaving home for good, leaving a big hole in our lives. As familiar emotional supports fall away, we can be left with a tremendous loss of focus and a sense of just drifting along through life.

Another distracting and emotionally unsettling life event is the hormonal shifts that occur during the "change of life"—menopause for women and andropause for men. While it is beyond the scope of this book to discuss the change of life for both genders, I do urge you to pass through it consciously and actively rather than passively, taking steps to cope with the symptoms. Some excellent books on the subject are *The Wisdom of Menopause* by Dr. Christiane Northrup, *The Andropause Mystery: Unravelling Truths about the Male Menopause* by Robert S. Tan, and *Male Menopause* and *The Whole Man Program* by Jed Diamond. Others can be found in the resource section at the back of this book.

2. Loss of Motivation

The second factor that can lead to a decline in performance is loss of motivation or passion for one's work. In midlife, some people find themselves in a "been-there-done-that" frame of mind where nothing seems new or fresh anymore. Whereas in the early part of their careers new and exciting challenges always seemed just around the corner, now work has become stale. It is no longer fun or challenging.

3. The Inability to Adapt

One of the main contributors to loss of motivation is the inability to adapt. As we get older and the technologies around us keep changing, there is a great temptation to just give up and stop learning. In the rapidly changing computer industry where there seems to be a faster, smarter computer system or software every couple of months, the joke among consultants is, "Let's not keep up." In other words, "What we know is good enough, so let's stop here."

Unfortunately, none of us has this luxury. As our fields develop and evolve, so must we. Nothing will kill motivation more quickly than becoming afraid of the unknown and resistant to change. For example, I know many middle-aged people who cannot cope with computers, E-mail, or the Internet, technologies that have become fundamental to the way we do business today. Their fear and unwillingness to learn make them appear stubborn and behind the times. While a certain amount of physiological aging does occur in the brain, we do not have to lose our ability to learn and adapt. Learning new technologies and ways of working goes a long way toward keeping us young and sharp.

4. Loss of Functional Health

Since people are living so long these days—an average of seventy-eight years for men and eighty-four years for women, we can no longer speak only of the life span, but must now consider the *health span,* how long a person can function at optimal levels of health. The goal of every man or woman must be to create a future of *compressed morbidity,* squeezing poor health and one's final illness into the shortest possible period at the end of one's life. No one can maintain a level of passion and motivation for their work if they are suffering from avoidable and debilitating diseases such as type 2 diabetes, heart disease, hypertension, obesity, and chronic fatigue.

5. Complacency

Our greatest enemy is becoming complacent about our jobs, our health, and our lives. It's easy to tell oneself: "I know enough about my job. What I know about my field has always been good enough to get by on. Why should I go to the inconvenience of getting on a plane and taking those company training seminars?" As we get older, there is always the temptation to become complacent.

To avoid complacency, one of the main questions you should ask yourself is: "What sort of a return am I getting on the time I invest in my work?" When we engage in nothing but low-risk activities and projects, we are likely to be getting back small returns. When we have the courage, the health profile, and the willingness to take on new challenges and to take some risks, the return we will get on our time is always greater. In turn, these greater returns generate greater energy and enthusiasm for taking more risks and becoming more productive.

Manage Your Performance for Career Extension

The secret to career extension is learning how to manage one's performance. While I myself cannot do the same things physically that I could do in my twenties, my health age is far lower than 99 percent of the men my age because my fitness levels are far greater. The energy and passion I bring to my work with athletes and the results we achieve together keep clients coming back for more. I have had to adjust my consulting and coaching tactics somewhat as I've gotten older, but the men and women I work with still respect me and are still in awe of the way that I follow my own principles regarding nutrition, exercise, lifestyle, and health. I do less work traveling around the country with athletes and sports teams now, and concentrate more on creating wellness and lifestyle programs in my hometown of New Orleans. And I continue to research cutting edge ways of serving the health needs of my clients.

To give you an example of how I apply the art of career extension to my clients, I want to tell you the story of twenty-year NFL veteran Morten Andersen, someone I've been working with since 1987. I can think of few people who have managed to sustain their motivation and passion for the job as well as Morten has. At forty-one, he has been playing longer than anyone else in the NFL, where the average career lasts about 3.2 years. He first played for the New Orleans Saints, then with the Atlanta Falcons and New York Giants, and as of this writing, with the Kansas City Chiefs. He's had a tremendous track record, has been to the Super Bowl, and is predicted to be elected to the NFL Hall of Fame in the near future. Morten's current goal is to play professional football until the age of fifty, something that has never been done before. But he also said in a recent article in the New Orleans *Times-Picayune,* "If I don't get to fifty, does that mean I've failed? No, it doesn't. It just means that I still had a pretty long career. I want to play as long as I'm enjoying it, and I'm enjoying it still. As long as I can be productive and kick well and produce."

Productivity and enjoyment—those are very key points to sustaining a career, whether you are an athlete or a lawyer or a stockbroker.

However, when Morten joined the Giants in 2001, for the first time in his life, he had to try out for his job because of his age. And this tryout might not be his last if he wants to last nine more seasons. Instead of being angry or discouraged about the tryout, Morten took it in stride:

I've never experienced anything like it before. . . . It was kind of interesting. I didn't come in and just sign a contract because I'm one of the best kickers in the country. I had to kick against Brad Daliuso and another kid from the arena football league. That was like going back to college for me, being a freshman in college and having to prove myself all over again. It kind of brought back the competitive spirit in me. You have to be realistic. I'm forty-one years old and I don't blame the Giants for wanting to look at what they're investing in. Kind of like, "Let's see if Grandpa can still kick 'em from fifty yards and still hit the kickoff." And I think I showed him I could. That's why I won the job.

Morten knows that an NFL kicker his age has to continually prove himself. And he does, time and time again.

Eight Ways to Sustain Your Motivation

In the fourteen years that Morten has been my client, he and I have conscientiously worked toward extending his career by keeping him motivated and on top of his form. Sustaining motivation for the lifetime of your career involves learning skills to keep you focused and fresh, cultivating a positive mental attitude, and staying on top of your health. Here are some essential strategies that I have discovered.

1. Enjoy What You Are Doing

Many people lose their focus because they don't enjoy the work they are doing. One of the most important reasons for Morten Andersen's career longevity long after others have retired is his love of football. "I want to play as long as I'm enjoying it and I'm really enjoying it still." If you can't find joy and fulfillment in what you do for a living, then you're not really living.

Finding enjoyment in your work can take many forms. Sometimes it involves shifting your focus onto an aspect of your field that is more exciting and rewarding for you. A client of mine spent thirteen years developing, writing, and editing books for major publishing houses. In the last year and a half, however, she found herself feeling burned out and bored in her job. She had earned degrees in writing at Columbia University and New York University because she wanted to become a writer but became a "book doctor" to pay the bills. Her real love was anthropology, and she had spent over a decade traveling the world, meeting people from the Mayan, African, Aztec, and Native American cultures.

She realized that if she was ever going to fulfill her ambition of sharing the unique knowledge she had gathered, she had to come up with a plan that would enable her to write her own books. She agreed to ghostwrite two projects, which would enable her to put aside enough money to take off six months to write her own book. In the meantime, she wrote a book proposal and sample chapter so that her literary agent could sell her own project. Now she is experiencing the joy and the challenges of doing her own creative work and creating strategies to help her publisher market it once it is published.

Feeling joy in what you do is one of the keys to sustaining motivation. Sometimes that means shifting the focus of your work to another area within your field. Other times it might mean doing a complete life evaluation and deciding to branch out into a new career. Or, like Morten Andersen, if you already love what you are doing, don't allow other people to tell you that you can't do it anymore. Fight for your right to do the work you love by learning how to manage your performance and energy.

One of the easiest ways to lose motivation is to believe that what you are doing is not productive. No one wants to think that their job doesn't really matter or that people do not care about their opinion.

One way to get a true gauge of the importance of your work is to *do a self-audit.*

- Sit down with a pencil and a piece of paper and be honest about all that you have done in the last six months to a year. You may be surprised at how much you have accomplished.
- Ask a trusted coworker or supervisor to give you some positive feedback on your contributions to the office for the last year or so.
- Be prepared to hear some constructive criticism that can help you to improve your overall performance. Choosing your adviser well—someone you trust and who looks fondly upon you—will take the sting out of the criticism.

Volunteer to help with work-related social activities such as dinners, parties, and fund-raisers. I was initially perceived at Elmwood Fitness as something of an outsider, working with the kind of world-class clients and athletes that I do. Some people found that very intimidating. I am also older than most of the young staff, who have all been together for many years. It wasn't until we were planning a party for our membership that this attitude changed. I asked them what I could do to help and then worked for seven straight hours, helping to plan and prepare for the party. After that, everyone looked upon me as "one of us."

Don't forget that there is a social aspect to the office and that promoting warmer human connections among the office staff is just as important as doing good business. People who know and respect one another on more than one level usually work together more efficiently. A staff that plays together stays together.

Look for ways to put meaning into your work, ways to feel that you are making a difference. One way to accomplish this is to do more of the type of work that you truly believe in or that truly helps you to grow in your career. This might mean asking to be transferred to a department that will make greater use of your skills (but be prepared to be challenged) or, if you are an entrepreneur, shifting the focus of your work to make it more creative or meaningful.

3. Prepare for the Challenge

As we have seen, there is a cultural expectation that when we get older, we are no longer up to the job. The only way to overcome this belief system is to be willing to prove yourself and consciously prepare for whatever challenges you must face.

Develop a positive mental attitude.

Always be prepared, whether you are getting ready to go up against the Young Turks in your office who want your job, win a new account, or lead your team to complete their project with record success. Learn all you can about the work you are doing, the new technologies in your industry, the market you are aiming for, the clients and coworkers on your team, and your competition.

4. Impress the Decision Makers

After Morten's tryout for the Giants, the coach said to me, "He's got a presence about him, a confidence. Morten is a perfectionist and a true professional." I too can see this quality in Morten. There are some guys that I send out onto the field with my fingers crossed, hoping they will make the grade. Not so with Morten Andersen. The man projects such an aura of authority and talent that you never doubt that he will turn in a fine performance.

Although the word *presence* evokes an almost magical quality, the people who possess it have put much skill, preparation, and hard work behind developing it. We most often see that type of charisma prominently displayed in public speakers, great leaders and teachers, and artistic performers of all kinds. These are the individuals to watch because they can teach us much about what it means to influence people through pure presence.

I have a forty-eight-year-old client, Joy, who used to be a professional singer in New York City. She left the field of music for eight years to pursue other interests but recently had an opportunity to make a comeback when she was invited to sing as part of a local concert series. Joy committed herself to singing some pretty challenging music. Once she began rehearsing, however, she discovered that the vocal skills that had been second nature to her when she was practicing for two or three hours daily were now very challenging. Her high notes were no longer full and effortless and her breath support and ability to sustain long musical phrases was shaky.

For a while she thought about giving up, since the first concert was in a month, but then she began asking herself what music really meant to her and what she was willing to do and to risk to be able to sing once more. She came to the conclusion that she passionately loved musical performance and was not willing to give it up, now that she had a second chance. But if she didn't impress the decision makers, the man running the concert series, and the public, her comeback would be over before it started. Her lack of confidence was exacerbated by the perfectionist performance standards her teachers and coaches in New York had placed upon her.

At that point she had an epiphany. "What if I just let go of the need for absolute perfection and sing for the pure joy of it, doing the absolute best I can? I know I've been well trained and can sell a song because I have the theatrical talent. And I know that I have a great voice." With these assets in mind, Joy made a commitment to enjoy the journey, to find out what music could mean in her present life.

As she practiced daily her voice and her upper range began to come back to her. She started to remember every bit of technique and every trick she'd ever learned and began utilizing them again. Most important, she realized that she had always been a crowd pleaser who enjoyed the challenge of getting up in front of an audience and interacting with their energy.

On the night of the concert, she was thoroughly prepared, dressed to the nines, and ready for whatever would come. Her performance was mesmerizing. Afterward, people came up to her and complimented her, saying that she had by far been the best performer that night. One woman told her, "My God, do you ever have a stage presence. Time stopped when you began to sing and the entire mood in the room completely changed. It was as if we were transported to another world."

Developing presence and impressing the decision makers happens when we love what we are doing, dedicate ourselves to performing as well as we possibly can, do everything within our power to prepare ourselves, and really learn how to communicate with the people with or for whom we are doing the job.

5. Take Care of Yourself

As I've said, it is possible to keep one's health age much lower than one's chronological age. In the fourteen years we have worked together, Morten Andersen has been concerned not just about his functional kicking or his training. He's also been concerned about his triglycerides, his body fat to lean muscle ratio, and so on—all the factors that will keep him strong, vital, and capable of doing his job. And when he finally retires, unlike a great many of the unhealthy and overweight players in the NFL, he will be able to enjoy his life and expect to live a long time in good health.

Taking care of yourself so that you can perform at your highest level involves managing four important factors:

- Mental attitude
- Overall health
- Nutrition
- Exercise

Most people do not realize that premature aging, disease, and fatigue are controlled 75 percent by your lifestyle. If you want not only to survive at your job but also to continue to advance, you must have a well-tuned body—your immune system, your cardiovascular system, and so on. When your physical health is in place and when you exercise regularly, you will quickly snap back from any setbacks that come your way.

I have a client, Alice, who overdid her workout in the gym because she wanted to look good for a presentation at work. Even though her back, which was her weakest link and the area we were working on, was giving her warning signs of strain, she kept going, pushing to do more and more sit-ups.

As the day progressed, Alice found that she was having more and more difficulty with muscle spasms in her lower back. By the time she returned home from her errands, she was unable to stand up straight and was experiencing pains that radiated into her abdominal area. She was in a panic, realizing that she might have sabotaged her presentation, which was due in a week, by overtraining.

Alice had several factors in her favor, however. I had taught her a great deal about nutrition, and she always ate foods that were good for her. She exercised faithfully and (at least most of the time) intelligently. She had also, with my help, developed a very good supplementation program.

Alice called her network chiropractor, a physician with whom she worked regularly and who knew her body very well, and set up appointments for the entire week. On my recommendation, she increased her doses of bovine colostrum to further strengthen her immune system, and began taking more MSM (methyl-sulfonyl-methane) to help repair her muscles and joints, the homeopathic remedy Arnica Montana to help repair muscle tissue, and an herbal supplement called Zyflamend to reduce inflammation and promote cell and joint repair. She also increased her protein intake by a few ounces a day because she knew that protein is the only nutrient that can repair damaged muscle tissue.

The next day she could stand up straight again even though she was very stiff and sore, could only walk with care, and could not take a deep breath without pain. She had another chiropractic treatment. The following day she was much improved, though still sore. By the third day, after another treatment, she felt well enough to realize that she was going to be able to make her presentation.

Her recovery time was phenomenal, and I was very proud of how intelligently she had managed it. When I asked her why she thought she was able to recover so quickly, she said, "I'm really clear that I could snap back like that only because I eat properly, exercise regularly, and take very good care of myself. When I hurt my back four years ago, I was down for weeks. After that, I knew I had to change my lifestyle, and I've been working on that ever since. This whole experience really proved to me what you always say, that maintaining good health is the key to performance. I truly surprised myself."

6. Overcome the Mind-set of the People Who See You As "Aging"

As we get older in a culture too easily impressed by youth, we must be willing to educate the people around us about the stamina, creativity, and greater vision of the experienced veteran. The best way to do this is to be fully present and at the height of our powers during times when the stakes are high and the heat is on.

The young person you are up against at the office may have skill, but he or she has never been tested. The older individual has both skill and experience. If you are willing to take care of your health and your mental focus and make a strong commitment to your work, you will always come out looking good.

Changing the mind-set of the people around you also involves a willingness to take risks—and even to fail once in a while. When Morten Andersen agreed to try out for the Giants, what if he hadn't made it? That wouldn't mean that he would never kick again, because he is a proven commodity. Another team would have called him three games into the season when one of their rookies folded.

7. Diversify—*Wisely*

One way to keep yourself motivated, your job interesting, and make yourself a more valuable employee is to diversify your skills. But you should never do this at the expense of losing touch with whatever got you to your present position in the first place. While learning new skills and diversifying your assets, don't forget to *maintain* the skills that put you on top.

When diversifying your skills, never forget why your company hired you. If your plan is to increase your motivation and performance by acquiring new skills, understand that you can't lose sight of the job description that got you to the top in the first place.

8. Remember That No Game Stays the Same Over Time

As the technologies and ways of doing business shift in this rapidly changing world, you must be able to develop flexibility. No matter what field you are in, things will inevitably change. If you have the vision, you will often see a change coming two steps down the road, or you may realize that *you and your objectives have changed.* Even though Joy pulled off a great performance, she realized that, at age forty-eight, she was no longer headed for the Metropolitan Opera. Nor did she want to go back to singing full-time. She is exploring new musical options she never would have considered before. Currently, she is developing a repertoire of blues songs and ballads so that she can sing in local clubs, resorts, and hotels. With her vocal technique, her ability to communicate with her audience, and her years of acting and theatrical training, she is light-years ahead of other singers out there who just have a pretty voice. Most important, she is thoroughly enjoying what she is doing.

The world around us and the careers we have chosen may change, but if we can keep alive our focus, our ability to adapt, our health, our passion, our enjoyment of what we do, and our commitment, we can sustain our motivation for a lifetime, always finding new frontiers and new challenges.

PART FOUR

The Optimum Performance Program

16

Your Twenty-one-Day
Optimum Performance
Program

This twenty-one-day program is meant to serve as a guide to help you get a strong start making the lifestyle changes described in this book. Following this program for three weeks will help you to create healthier routines and to make them a part of your daily life. You should also begin to feel changes in your life, such as more energy, a greater capacity for focus and performance, increased strength and aerobic capacity, better digestion, more peace of mind, and a restful night's sleep.

Don't be discouraged if you don't accomplish every task every day, or if you don't make every meal nutritionally perfect. The important thing is to improve, to make steady progress in substituting good habits for ones that do not serve your health and well-being.

Once you have made all of these changes a permanent part of your lifestyle, you will continue to see amazing improvements. A few things to remember:

- *Reevaluate your caloric needs.* As your scale weight drops and your body fat decreases, you will periodically—about once a month—need to go back and recalculate how many calories you need per day. A thinner, leaner body needs fewer calories for metabolic efficiency.

- *Manage your stress levels.* Stress is a major energy thief. Use tools such as visualizations, meditations, and exercise to keep your stress under control.
- *Keep your exercise program changing as your body changes.* As your strength and endurance increase continue to add weights and exercises according to the instructions in chapter 13.

To begin, I'd like you to photocopy the following training log. Take a moment at the end of each day to check off each statement with a plus (+) or a minus (−). Your ultimate goal is a perfect score of twenty points.

Training Log

____ I ate three nutritious meals and two or three snacks today.

____ I chose only lean protein sources.

____ I chose complex carbohydrates over simple sugars.

____ I ate at least 25 grams of a high-fiber foods such as oatmeal or a bran muffin.

____ I had at least five servings of vegetables today.

____ I had at least two servings of fruit today.

____ I avoided saturated fats and ate healthy unsaturated fats.

____ I enjoyed soy protein powder as one of my snacks.

____ I drank between ½ to 1 ounce of water per pound of body weight.

____ I did not have more than two cups of coffee or tea.

____ I avoided soft drinks containing sugar and caffeine.

____ I did not allow more than three or four hours between meals and snacks.

____ I understand that desserts are a special treat, so I skipped mine today.

____ I took my supplements.

____ I did not eat after eight at night.

____ I did either the Pro Circuit today or at least twenty minutes of aerobic exercise.

____ I used visualization to help me solve problems and handle stress.

____ I did at least two one-minute meditations today to keep myself focused and relaxed.

_____ I did at least one ten- to twenty-minute meditation.

_____ If needed, I sought guidance or perspective from a trusted mentor or friend.

Day 1
Nutrition
(Use the Guidelines for Eating and the Meal Plans in chapter 10 as a guide. Also include what *time* you eat each meal.)

Breakfast _____

Snack _____

Lunch _____

Snack _____

Dinner _____

Snack _____

Daily fluid intake. Aim for ½ to 1 ounce per pound of body weight. Example, if you weigh 160 pounds, you should drink between 1½ to 3 1.5-liter bottles of water. _____

Coffee, tea, sodas. Always drink in moderation, since these contain caffeine and sugar. Most of your daily fluid intake should be water.

_____

Stress Management
Time spent meditating or doing visualizations _____

Number of one-minute meditations _____

Time spent journaling or doing a self-audit _____

Daily Exercise
(Don't forget to warm up and cool down for 10 minutes!)
Time spent doing Pro Circuit workout (20, 30, or 45 minutes) _____

_____

Time spent moving to another exercise station (beginner—15 seconds, intermediate—10 seconds, advanced—5 seconds) _____

Number of circuits completed _____

Target heart-rate zone _____ bpm. I stayed in my zone (always, mostly) _____

How I felt at the end of my workout _____

_____

End-of-the-Day Evaluation

Type of sleep (restful, restless) _____ . How many hours _____

Stress levels (high, medium, low) _____

Overall productivity levels (high, medium, low) _____

Level of energy (high, medium, low) _____

Significant accomplishments _____

_____

_____

Day 2

Nutrition

(Use the Guidelines for Eating and the Meal Plans in chapter 10 as a guide. Also include what *time* you eat each meal.)

Breakfast _____

Snack _____

Lunch _____

Snack _____

Dinner _____

Snack _____

Daily fluid intake. Aim for ½ to 1 ounce per pound of body weight. Example, if you weigh 160 pounds, you should drink between 1½ to 3 1.5-liter bottles of water. _____

Coffee, tea, sodas. Always drink in moderation, since these contain caffeine and sugar. Most of your daily fluid intake should be water.

_____

Stress Management

Time spent meditating or doing visualizations _____

Number of one-minute meditations _____

Time spent journaling or doing a self-audit _____

Daily Exercise
(Don't forget to warm up and cool down for 10 minutes!)

Time spent doing aerobic exercise (20, 30, or 45 minutes) _____

Type of aerobic exercise (walking, bicycling, jogging, step class, etc.)

_____

Target heart-rate zone _____ bpm. I stayed in my zone (always, mostly) _____

How I felt at the end of my workout _____

_____

End-of-the-Day Evaluation

Type of sleep (restful, restless) _____ . How many hours _____

Stress levels (high, medium, low) _____

Overall productivity levels (high, medium, low) _____

Level of energy (high, medium, low) _____

Significant accomplishments _____

_____

_____

Day 3

Nutrition

(Use the Guidelines for Eating and the Meal Plans in chapter 10 as a guide. Also include what *time* you eat each meal.)

Breakfast _____

Snack _____

Lunch _____

Snack _____

Dinner _____

Snack _____

Daily fluid intake. Aim for ½ to 1 ounce per pound of body weight. Example, if you weigh 160 pounds, you should drink between 1½ to 3 1.5-liter bottles of water. _____

Coffee, tea, sodas. Always drink in moderation, since these contain caffeine and sugar. Most of your daily fluid intake should be water.

_____

Stress Management

Time spent meditating or doing visualizations _____

Number of one-minute meditations _____

Time spent journaling or doing a self-audit _____

Daily Exercise
(Don't forget to warm up and cool down for 10 minutes!)
Time spent doing Pro Circuit workout (20, 30, or 45 minutes) _____

_____

Time spent moving to another exercise station (beginner—15 seconds, intermediate—10 seconds, advanced—5 seconds) _____

Number of circuits completed _____

Target heart-rate zone _____ bpm. I stayed in my zone (always, mostly) _____

How I felt at the end of my workout _____

_____

End-of-the-Day Evaluation
Type of sleep (restful, restless) _____ . How many hours _____

Stress levels (high, medium, low) _____

Overall productivity levels (high, medium, low) _____

Level of energy (high, medium, low) _____

Significant accomplishments _____

_____

_____

Day 4

Nutrition
(Use the Guidelines for Eating and the Meal Plans in chapter 10 as a guide. Also include what *time* you eat each meal.)

Breakfast _____

Snack _____

Lunch _____

Snack _____

Dinner _____

Snack _____

Daily fluid intake. Aim for ½ to 1 ounce per pound of body weight. Example, if you weigh 160 pounds, you should drink between 1½ to 3 1.5-liter bottles of water. _____

Coffee, tea, sodas. Always drink in moderation, since these contain caffeine and sugar. Most of your daily fluid intake should be water.

_____

Stress Management

Time spent meditating or doing visualizations _____

Number of one-minute meditations _____

Time spent journaling or doing a self-audit _____

Daily Exercise
(Don't forget to warm up and cool down for 10 minutes!)
Time spent doing aerobic exercise (20, 30, or 45 minutes) _____

Type of aerobic exercise (walking, bicycling, jogging, step class, etc.)
_____

Target heart-rate zone _____ bpm. I stayed in my zone (always, mostly) _____

How I felt at the end of my workout _____
_____

End-of-the-Day Evaluation

Type of sleep (restful, restless) _____ . How many hours _____

Stress levels (high, medium, low) _____

Overall productivity levels (high, medium, low) _____

Level of energy (high, medium, low) _____

Significant accomplishments _____
_____
_____

Day 5

Nutrition
(Use the Guidelines for Eating and the Meal Plans in chapter 10 as a guide. Also include what *time* you eat each meal.)

Breakfast _____

Snack _____

Lunch _____

Snack _____

Dinner _____

Snack _____

Daily fluid intake. Aim for ½ to 1 ounce per pound of body weight. Example, if you weigh 160 pounds, you should drink between 1½ to 3 1.5-liter bottles of water. _____

Coffee, tea, sodas. Always drink in moderation, since these contain caffeine and sugar. Most of your daily fluid intake should be water.

___

Stress Management

Time spent meditating or doing visualizations _____

Number of one-minute meditations _____

Time spent journaling or doing a self-audit _____

Daily Exercise
(Don't forget to warm up and cool down for 10 minutes!)
Time spent doing Pro Circuit workout (20, 30, or 45 minutes) _____

___

Time spent moving to another exercise station (beginner—15 seconds, intermediate—10 seconds, advanced—5 seconds) _____

Number of circuits completed _____

Target heart-rate zone _____ bpm. I stayed in my zone (always, mostly) _____

How I felt at the end of my workout _____

___

End-of-the-Day Evaluation

Type of sleep (restful, restless) _____ . How many hours _____

Stress levels (high, medium, low) _____

Overall productivity levels (high, medium, low) _____

Level of energy (high, medium, low) _____

Significant accomplishments _____

___

___

Day 6

Nutrition
(Use the Guidelines for Eating and the Meal Plans in chapter 10 as a guide. Also include what *time* you eat each meal.)

Breakfast _____

Snack _____

Lunch _____

Snack _____

Dinner _____

Snack _____

Daily fluid intake. Aim for ½ to 1 ounce per pound of body weight. Example, if you weigh 160 pounds, you should drink between 1½ to 3 1.5-liter bottles of water. _____

Coffee, tea, sodas. Always drink in moderation, since these contain caffeine and sugar. Most of your daily fluid intake should be water.

Stress Management

Time spent meditating or doing visualizations _____

Number of one-minute meditations _____

Time spent journaling or doing a self-audit _____

Daily Exercise
(Don't forget to warm up and cool down for 10 minutes!)

Time spent doing aerobic exercise (20, 30, or 45 minutes) _____

Type of aerobic exercise (walking, bicycling, jogging, step class, etc.)
_____

Target heart-rate zone _____ bpm. I stayed in my zone (always, mostly) _____

How I felt at the end of my workout _____
_____

_____

End-of-the-Day Evaluation

Type of sleep (restful, restless) _____ . How many hours _____

Stress levels (high, medium, low) _____

Overall productivity levels (high, medium, low) _____

Level of energy (high, medium, low) _____

Significant accomplishments _____
_____

_____

_____

Day 7

Nutrition

(Use the Guidelines for Eating and the Meal Plans in chapter 10 as a guide. Also include what *time* you eat each meal.)

Breakfast _____

Snack _____

Lunch _____

Snack _____

Dinner _____

Snack _____

Daily fluid intake. Aim for ½ to 1 ounce per pound of body weight. Example, if you weigh 160 pounds, you should drink between 1½ to 3 1.5-liter bottles of water. _____

Coffee, tea, sodas. Always drink in moderation, since these contain caffeine and sugar. Most of your daily fluid intake should be water.

_____

Stress Management

Time spent meditating or doing visualizations _____

Number of one-minute meditations _____

Time spent journaling or doing a self-audit _____

Daily Exercise

(Take a day off to rest and rejuvenate.)

End-of-the-Day Evaluation

Type of sleep (restful, restless) _____ . How many hours _____

Stress levels (high, medium, low) _____

Overall productivity levels (high, medium, low) _____

Level of energy (high, medium, low) _____

Significant accomplishments _____

_____

_____

_____

Day 8

Nutrition

(Use the Guidelines for Eating and the Meal Plans in chapter 10 as a guide. Also include what *time* you eat each meal.)

Breakfast _____

Snack _____

Lunch _____

Snack _____

Dinner _____

Snack _____

Daily fluid intake. Aim for ½ to 1 ounce per pound of body weight. Example, if you weigh 160 pounds, you should drink between 1½ to 3 1.5-liter bottles of water. _____

Coffee, tea, sodas. Always drink in moderation, since these contain caffeine and sugar. Most of your daily fluid intake should be water.

_____

Stress Management

Time spent meditating or doing visualizations _____

Number of one-minute meditations _____

Time spent journaling or doing a self-audit _____

Daily Exercise
(Don't forget to warm up and cool down for 10 minutes!)

Time spent doing Pro Circuit workout (20, 30, or 45 minutes) _____

_____

Time spent moving to another exercise station (beginner—15 seconds, intermediate—10 seconds, advanced—5 seconds) _____

Number of circuits completed _____

Target heart-rate zone _____ bpm. I stayed in my zone (always, mostly) _____

How I felt at the end of my workout _____

_____

End-of-the-Day Evaluation

Type of sleep (restful, restless) _____ . How many hours _____

Stress levels (high, medium, low) _____

Overall productivity levels (high, medium, low) _____

Level of energy (high, medium, low) _____

Significant accomplishments _____

_____

_____

Day 9

Nutrition

(Use the Guidelines for Eating and the Meal Plans in chapter 10 as a guide. Also include what *time* you eat each meal.)

Breakfast _____

Snack _____

Lunch _____

Snack _____

Dinner _____

Snack _____

Daily fluid intake. Aim for ½ to 1 ounce per pound of body weight. Example, if you weigh 160 pounds, you should drink between 1½ to 3 1.5-liter bottles of water. _____

Coffee, tea, sodas. Always drink in moderation, since these contain caffeine and sugar. Most of your daily fluid intake should be water.

_____

Stress Management

Time spent meditating or doing visualizations _____

Number of one-minute meditations _____

Time spent journaling or doing a self-audit _____

Daily Exercise
(Don't forget to warm up and cool down for 10 minutes!)

Time spent doing aerobic exercise (20, 30, or 45 minutes) _____

Type of aerobic exercise (walking, bicycling, jogging, step class, etc.)

_____

Target heart-rate zone _____ bpm. I stayed in my zone (always, mostly) _____

How I felt at the end of my workout _____

_____

End-of-the-Day Evaluation

Type of sleep (restful, restless) _____ . How many hours _____

Stress levels (high, medium, low) _____

Overall productivity levels (high, medium, low) _____

Level of energy (high, medium, low) _____

Significant accomplishments _____

_____

_____

Day 10

Nutrition

(Use the Guidelines for Eating and the Meal Plans in chapter 10 as a guide. Also include what *time* you eat each meal.)

Breakfast _____

Snack _____

Lunch _____

Snack _____

Dinner _____

Snack _____

Stress Management

Time spent meditating or doing visualizations _____

Number of one-minute meditations _____

Time spent journaling or doing a self-audit _____

Daily Exercise
(Don't forget to warm up and cool down for 10 minutes!)

Time spent doing Pro Circuit workout (20, 30, or 45 minutes) _____

_____

Time spent moving to another exercise station (beginner—15 seconds, intermediate—10 seconds, advanced—5 seconds) _____

Number of circuits completed _____

Target heart-rate zone _____ bpm. I stayed in my zone (always, mostly) _____

How I felt at the end of my workout _____

_____

End-of-the-Day Evaluation

Type of sleep (restful, restless) _____ . How many hours _____

Stress levels (high, medium, low) _____

Overall productivity levels (high, medium, low) _____

Level of energy (high, medium, low) _____

Significant accomplishments _____

_____

_____

Day 11

Nutrition

(Use the Guidelines for Eating and the Meal Plans in chapter 10 as a guide. Also include what *time* you eat each meal.)

Breakfast _____

Snack _____

Lunch _____

Snack _____

Dinner _____

Snack _____

Daily fluid intake. Aim for ½ to 1 ounce per pound of body weight. Example, if you weigh 160 pounds, you should drink between 1½ to 3 1.5-liter bottles of water. _____

Coffee, tea, sodas. Always drink in moderation, since these contain caffeine and sugar. Most of your daily fluid intake should be water.

_____

Stress Management

Time spent meditating or doing visualizations _____

Number of one-minute meditations _____

Time spent journaling or doing a self-audit _____

Daily Exercise
(Don't forget to warm up and cool down for 10 minutes!)

Time spent doing aerobic exercise (20, 30, or 45 minutes) _____

Type of aerobic exercise (walking, bicycling, jogging, step class, etc.)

_____

Target heart-rate zone _____ bpm. I stayed in my zone (always, mostly) _____

How I felt at the end of my workout _____

_____

End-of-the-Day Evaluation

Type of sleep (restful, restless) _____ . How many hours _____

Stress levels (high, medium, low) _____

Overall productivity levels (high, medium, low) _____

Level of energy (high, medium, low) _____

Significant accomplishments _____

_____

_____

Day 12

Nutrition

(Use the Guidelines for Eating and the Meal Plans in chapter 10 as a guide. Also include what *time* you eat each meal.)

Breakfast _____

Snack _____

Lunch _____

Snack _____

Dinner _____

Snack _____

Daily fluid intake. Aim for ½ to 1 ounce per pound of body weight. Example, if you weigh 160 pounds, you should drink between 1½ to 3 1.5-liter bottles of water. _____

Coffee, tea, sodas. Always drink in moderation, since these contain caffeine and sugar. Most of your daily fluid intake should be water.

_____

Stress Management

Time spent meditating or doing visualizations _____

Number of one-minute meditations _____

Time spent journaling or doing a self-audit _____

Daily Exercise
(Don't forget to warm up and cool down for 10 minutes!)
Time spent doing Pro Circuit workout (20, 30, or 45 minutes) _____

_____

Time spent moving to another exercise station (beginner—15 seconds, intermediate—10 seconds, advanced—5 seconds) _____

Number of circuits completed _____

Target heart-rate zone _____ bpm. I stayed in my zone (always, mostly) _____

How I felt at the end of my workout _____

_____

End-of-the-Day Evaluation
Type of sleep (restful, restless) _____ . How many hours _____

Stress levels (high, medium, low) _____

Overall productivity levels (high, medium, low) _____

Level of energy (high, medium, low) _____

Significant accomplishments _____

_____

_____

Day 13

Nutrition
(Use the Guidelines for Eating and the Meal Plans in chapter 10 as a guide. Also include what *time* you eat each meal.)

Breakfast _____

Snack _____

Lunch _____

Snack _____

Dinner _____

Snack _____

Daily fluid intake. Aim for ½ to 1 ounce per pound of body weight. Example, if you weigh 160 pounds, you should drink between 1½ to 3 1.5-liter bottles of water. _____

Coffee, tea, sodas. Always drink in moderation, since these contain caffeine and sugar. Most of your daily fluid intake should be water.

_____

Stress Management

Time spent meditating or doing visualizations _____

Number of one-minute meditations _____

Time spent journaling or doing a self-audit _____

Daily Exercise
(Don't forget to warm up and cool down for 10 minutes!)

Time spent doing aerobic exercise (20, 30, or 45 minutes) _____

Type of aerobic exercise (walking, bicycling, jogging, step class, etc.)

_____

Target heart-rate zone _____ bpm. I stayed in my zone (always, mostly) _____

How I felt at the end of my workout _____

_____

End-of-the-Day Evaluation

Type of sleep (restful, restless) _____ . How many hours _____

Stress levels (high, medium, low) _____

Overall productivity levels (high, medium, low) _____

Level of energy (high, medium, low) _____

Significant accomplishments _____

_____

_____

Day 14

Nutrition

(Use the Guidelines for Eating and the Meal Plans in chapter 10 as a guide. Also include what *time* you eat each meal.)

Breakfast _____

Snack _____

Lunch _____

Snack _____

Dinner _____

Snack _____

Daily fluid intake. Aim for ½ to 1 ounce per pound of body weight. Example, if you weigh 160 pounds, you should drink between 1½ to 3 1.5-liter bottles of water. _____

Coffee, tea, sodas. Always drink in moderation, since these contain caffeine and sugar. Most of your daily fluid intake should be water.

Stress Management

Time spent meditating or doing visualizations _____

Number of one-minute meditations _____

Time spent journaling or doing a self-audit _____

Daily Exercise

(Take a day off to rest and rejuvenate.)

End-of-the-Day Evaluation

Type of sleep (restful, restless) _____ . How many hours _____

Stress levels (high, medium, low) _____

Overall productivity levels (high, medium, low) _____

Level of energy (high, medium, low) _____

Significant accomplishments _____

_____

_____

Day 15

Nutrition

(Use the Guidelines for Eating and the Meal Plans in chapter 10 as a guide. Also include what *time* you eat each meal.)

Breakfast _____

Snack _____

Lunch _____

Snack _____

Dinner _____

Snack _____

Daily fluid intake. Aim for ½ to 1 ounce per pound of body weight. Example, if you weigh 160 pounds, you should drink between 1½ to 3 1.5-liter bottles of water. _____

Coffee, tea, sodas. Always drink in moderation, since these contain caffeine and sugar. Most of your daily fluid intake should be water.

Stress Management

Time spent meditating or doing visualizations _____

Number of one-minute meditations _____

Time spent journaling or doing a self-audit _____

Daily Exercise
(Don't forget to warm up and cool down for 10 minutes!)
Time spent doing Pro Circuit workout (20, 30, or 45 minutes) _____

_____

Time spent moving to another exercise station (beginner—15 seconds, intermediate—10 seconds, advanced—5 seconds) _____

Number of circuits completed _____

Target heart-rate zone _____ bpm. I stayed in my zone (always, mostly) _____

How I felt at the end of my workout _____

_____

End-of-the-Day Evaluation

Type of sleep (restful, restless) _____ . How many hours _____

Stress levels (high, medium, low) _____

Overall productivity levels (high, medium, low) _____

Level of energy (high, medium, low) _____

Significant accomplishments _____

_____

_____

Day 16

Nutrition
(Use the Guidelines for Eating and the Meal Plans in chapter 10 as a guide. Also include what *time* you eat each meal.)

Breakfast _____

Snack _____

Lunch _____

Snack _____

Dinner _____

Snack _____

Daily fluid intake. Aim for ½ to 1 ounce per pound of body weight. Example, if you weigh 160 pounds, you should drink between 1½ to 3 1.5-liter bottles of water. _____

Coffee, tea, sodas. Always drink in moderation, since these contain caffeine and sugar. Most of your daily fluid intake should be water.

Stress Management

Time spent meditating or doing visualizations _____

Number of one-minute meditations _____

Time spent journaling or doing a self-audit _____

Daily Exercise
(Don't forget to warm up and cool down for 10 minutes!)
Time spent doing aerobic exercise (20, 30, or 45 minutes) _____

Type of aerobic exercise (walking, bicycling, jogging, step class, etc.)

Target heart-rate zone _____ bpm. I stayed in my zone (always, mostly) _____

How I felt at the end of my workout _____

End-of-the-Day Evaluation

Type of sleep (restful, restless) _____ . How many hours _____

Stress levels (high, medium, low) _____

Overall productivity levels (high, medium, low) _____

Level of energy (high, medium, low) _____

Significant accomplishments _____

Day 17

Nutrition

(Use the Guidelines for Eating and the Meal Plans in chapter 10 as a guide. Also include what *time* you eat each meal.)

Breakfast _____

Snack _____

Lunch _____

Snack _____

Dinner _____

Snack _____

Daily fluid intake. Aim for ½ to 1 ounce per pound of body weight. Example, if you weigh 160 pounds, you should drink between 1½ to 3 1.5-liter bottles of water. _____

Coffee, tea, sodas. Always drink in moderation, since these contain caffeine and sugar. Most of your daily fluid intake should be water.

Stress Management

Time spent meditating or doing visualizations _____

Number of one-minute meditations _____

Time spent journaling or doing a self-audit _____

Daily Exercise
(Don't forget to warm up and cool down for 10 minutes!)

Time spent doing Pro Circuit workout (20, 30, or 45 minutes) _____

Time spent moving to another exercise station (beginner—15 seconds, intermediate—10 seconds, advanced—5 seconds) _____

Number of circuits completed _____

Target heart-rate zone _____ bpm. I stayed in my zone (always, mostly) _____

How I felt at the end of my workout _____

End-of-the-Day Evaluation

Type of sleep (restful, restless) _____ . How many hours _____

Stress levels (high, medium, low) _____

Overall productivity levels (high, medium, low) _____

Level of energy (high, medium, low) _____

Significant accomplishments _____

Day 18

Nutrition

(Use the Guidelines for Eating and the Meal Plans in chapter 10 as a guide. Also include what *time* you eat each meal.)

Breakfast _____

Snack _____

Lunch _____

Snack _____

Dinner _____

Snack _____

Daily fluid intake. Aim for ½ to 1 ounce per pound of body weight. Example, if you weigh 160 pounds, you should drink between 1½ to 3 1.5-liter bottles of water. _____

Coffee, tea, sodas. Always drink in moderation, since these contain caffeine and sugar. Most of your daily fluid intake should be water.

_____

Stress Management

Time spent meditating or doing visualizations _____

Number of one-minute meditations _____

Time spent journaling or doing a self-audit _____

Daily Exercise
(Don't forget to warm up and cool down for 10 minutes!)
Time spent doing aerobic exercise (20, 30, or 45 minutes) _____

Type of aerobic exercise (walking, bicycling, jogging, step class, etc.)

_____

Target heart-rate zone _____ bpm. I stayed in my zone (always, mostly) _____

How I felt at the end of my workout _____

_____

End-of-the-Day Evaluation
Type of sleep (restful, restless) _____. How many hours _____

Stress levels (high, medium, low) _____

Overall productivity levels (high, medium, low) _____

Level of energy (high, medium, low) _____

Significant accomplishments _____

_____

_____

Day 19

Nutrition

(Use the Guidelines for Eating and the Meal Plans in chapter 10 as a guide. Also include what *time* you eat each meal.)

Breakfast _____

Snack _____

Lunch _____

Snack _____

Dinner _____

Snack _____

Daily fluid intake. Aim for ½ to 1 ounce per pound of body weight. Example, if you weigh 160 pounds, you should drink between 1½ to 3 1.5-liter bottles of water. _____

Coffee, tea, sodas. Always drink in moderation, since these contain caffeine and sugar. Most of your daily fluid intake should be water.

_____

Stress Management

Time spent meditating or doing visualizations _____

Number of one-minute meditations _____

Time spent journaling or doing a self-audit _____

Daily Exercise
(Don't forget to warm up and cool down for 10 minutes!)

Time spent doing Pro Circuit workout (20, 30, or 45 minutes) _____

_____

Time spent moving to another exercise station (beginner—15 seconds, intermediate—10 seconds, advanced—5 seconds) _____

Number of circuits completed _____

Target heart-rate zone _____ bpm. I stayed in my zone (always, mostly) _____

How I felt at the end of my workout _____

_____

End-of-the-Day Evaluation

Type of sleep (restful, restless) _____ . How many hours _____

Stress levels (high, medium, low) _____

Overall productivity levels (high, medium, low) _____

Level of energy (high, medium, low) _____

Significant accomplishments _____

_____

_____

Day 20

Nutrition

(Use the Guidelines for Eating and the Meal Plans in chapter 10 as a guide. Also include what *time* you eat each meal.)

Breakfast _____

Snack _____

Lunch _____

Snack _____

Dinner _____

Snack _____

Daily fluid intake. Aim for ½ to 1 ounce per pound of body weight. Example, if you weigh 160 pounds, you should drink between 1½ to 3 1.5-liter bottles of water. _____

Coffee, tea, sodas. Always drink in moderation, since these contain caffeine and sugar. Most of your daily fluid intake should be water.

_____

Stress Management

Time spent meditating or doing visualizations _____

Number of one-minute meditations _____

Time spent journaling or doing a self-audit _____

Daily Exercise
(Don't forget to warm up and cool down for 10 minutes!)

Time spent doing aerobic exercise (20, 30, or 45 minutes) _____

Type of aerobic exercise (walking, bicycling, jogging, step class, etc.)

_____

Target heart-rate zone _____ bpm. I stayed in my zone (always, mostly) _____

How I felt at the end of my workout _____

_____

End-of-the-Day Evaluation

Type of sleep (restful, restless) _____ . How many hours _____

Stress levels (high, medium, low) _____

Overall productivity levels (high, medium, low) _____

Level of energy (high, medium, low) _____

Significant accomplishments _____

_____

_____

Day 21

Nutrition

(Use the Guidelines for Eating and the Meal Plans in chapter 10 as a guide. Also include what *time* you eat each meal.)

Breakfast _____

Snack _____

Lunch _____

Snack _____

Dinner _____

Snack _____

Daily fluid intake. Aim for ½ to 1 ounce per pound of body weight. Example, if you weigh 160 pounds, you should drink between 1½ to 3 1.5-liter bottles of water. _____

Coffee, tea, sodas. Always drink in moderation, since these contain caffeine and sugar. Most of your daily fluid intake should be water.

_____

Stress Management

Time spent meditating or doing visualizations _____

Number of one-minute meditations _____

Time spent journaling or doing a self-audit _____

Daily Exercise
(Take a day off to rest and rejuvenate.)

End-of-the-Day Evaluation

Type of sleep (restful, restless) _____ . How many hours _____

Stress levels (high, medium, low) _____

Overall productivity levels (high, medium, low) _____

Level of energy (high, medium, low) _____

Significant accomplishments _____

_____

_____

Appendix: A Ten-Year Risk Evaluation for Men and Women

For those readers who would like to get more specific about their risk factors according to what stage of life they are in (divided into five- to ten-year intervals), I have included a Ten-Year Risk Evaluation for both men and women. The goal of this questionnaire is to first look at the number of points allowed for health in your age group, then rate your total cholesterol, HDL, systolic blood pressure, and smoking profile (smoker or nonsmoker). Then simply add up your points and look at the final table to see how much of a risk you have for heart disease or a major event such as a heart attack within the next ten years. This questionnaire was published by the National Institute of Health in May of 2001.

Estimate of Ten-Year Risk for Men

Age	Points
20–34	–9
35–39	–4
40–44	0
45–49	3
50–54	6
55–59	8
60–64	10
65–69	11
70–74	12
75–79	13

Your points ____

TOTAL CHOLESTEROL

Total Cholesterol	Age 20–39	Age 40–49	Age 50–59	Age 60–69	Age 70–79
< 160	0	0	0	0	0
160–199	4	3	2	1	0
200–239	7	5	3	1	0
240–279	9	6	4	2	1
≥ 280	11	8	5	3	1

Your points ____

HDL

HDL (mg/dl)	Points
≥ 60	–1
50–59	0
40–49	1
< 40	2

Your points ____

NONSMOKER/SMOKER

	Age 20–39	Age 40–49	Age 50–59	Age 60–69	Age 70–79
Nonsmoker	0	0	0	0	0
Smoker	8	5	3	1	1

Your points ____

SYSTOLIC BLOOD PRESSURE

Systolic Blood Pressure (mmHg)	If Untreated	If Treated
< 120	0	0
120–129	0	1
130–139	1	2
140–159	1	2
≥ 160	2	3

Your points ____

TOTAL POINTS FOR MEN

Point Total	10-Year Risk %
< 0	< 1
0	1
1	1
2	1
3	1
4	1
5	2
6	2
7	3
8	4
9	5
10	6
11	8
12	10
13	12
14	16
15	20
16	25
≥ 17	≥ 30

Ten-year risk = _____ percent

Estimate of Ten-Year Risk for Women

Age	Points
20–34	–7
35–39	–3
40–44	0
45–49	3
50–54	6
55–59	8
60–64	10
65–69	12
70–74	14
75–79	16

Your points ____

TOTAL CHOLESTEROL

Total Cholesterol	Age 20–39	Age 40–49	Age 50–59	Age 60–69	Age 70–79
< 160	0	0	0	0	0
160–199	4	3	2	1	1
200–239	8	6	4	2	1
240–279	11	8	5	3	2
≥ 280	13	10	7	4	2

Your points ____

HDL

HDL (mg/dl)	Points
≥ 60	–1
50–59	0
40–49	1
< 40	2

Your points ____

NONSMOKER/SMOKER

	Age 20–39	Age 40–49	Age 50–59	Age 60–69	Age 70–79
Nonsmoker	0	0	0	0	0
Smoker	9	7	4	2	1

Your points ____

SYSTOLIC BLOOD PRESSURE

Systolic Blood Pressure (mmHg)	If Untreated	If Treated
< 120	0	0
120–129	1	3
130–139	2	4
140–159	3	5
≥ 160	4	6

Your points ____

TOTAL POINTS FOR WOMEN

Point Total	10-Year Risk %
< 9	< 1
9	1
10	1
11	1
12	1
13	2
14	2
15	3
16	4
17	5
18	6
19	8
20	11
21	14
22	17
23	22
24	27
≥ 25	≥ 30

Ten-year risk = _____ percent

Once you have completed this evaluation, look at the areas where you are strongest and those where you are weakest and use the tools in this book to improve your risk factors.

Resources to Help You

Medical Organizations

American Academy of Family
Physicians
11400 Tomahawk Creek Parkway
Leawood, KS 66211-2672
www.familydoctor.org

American Heart Association (AHA)
National Center
7272 Greenville Avenue
Dallas, TX 75231
800-242-8721
www.americanheart.org

Centers for Disease Control and
Prevention
National Center for Chronic Disease
Prevention and Health
Promotion
Division of Nutrition and Physical
Activity
4770 Buford Highway NE
Atlanta, GA 303421
770-488-5820
www.cdc.gov/nccdphp/dnpa

National Cholesterol Education
Program
NHLBI Health Information Center
P.O. Box 30105
Bethesda, MD 20824–0105
301-592-8573

Nutrition

American Dietetic Association (ADA)
216 West Jackson Boulevard
Chicago, IL 60606-6995
800-877-1600; 312-899-0040;
312-899-4739 (FAX)
800-366-1655 (Consumer Hotline)

E-mails: hotline@eatright.org;
infocenter@eatright.org

American Society for Clinical
Nutrition (ASCN)
9650 Rockville Pike
Bethesda, MD 20814
301-530-7110; 301-571-1863 (FAX)
E-mail: secretar@acsn.faseb.org

The Glycemic Research Institute
601 Pennsylvania Avenue, NW,
Suite 900
Washington, D.C. 20004
202-434-8270
www.glycemic.com
www.anndeweesallen.com

Personal Edge Performance Nutrition
Personal Edge Nutrition Products
P.O. Box 88940
St. Louis, MO 63188
888-982-EDGE (toll free)
www.personaledgeprotein.com

U.S. Food and Drug Administration
5600 Fishers Lane
Rockville, MD 20857-0001
888-463-6332
www.fda.gov

Fitness Organizations

American College of Sports Medicine
(ACSM)
401 W. Michigan Street
Indianapolis, IN 46206-3233
317-637-9200
www.acsm.org

American Council on Exercise (ACE)
5820 Oberlin Drive, Suite 102
San Diego, CA 92121-3787
619-535-8227
www.acefitness.org

Cooper Institute for Aerobic
   Research (CIAR)
12330 Preston Road
Dallas, TX 75230
214-701-8001
www.cooperinst.org

HeartMath LLC
14700 West Park Avenue
Boulder Creek, California 95006
800-450-9111; 831-338-8700

President's Council
   on Physical Fitness and Sports
Room 738-H Hubert H. Humphrey
   Building

200 Independence Avenue, SW
Washington, D.C. 20201-0004
www.fitness.gov

Shape Up America!
6707 Democracy Boulevard, Suite 306
Bethesda, MD 20817
301-493-5368
www.shapeup.org

The National Women's Health
   Information Center
8550 Arlington Boulevard, Suite 300
Fairfax, VA 22031
800-994-9662
800-220-5446 (TDD)
www.4woman.gov/faq/heartdis.htm

Books

Good Fat, Bad Fat: How to Lower Your Cholesterol and Reduce the Odds of a Heart Attack by William P. Castelli, M.D. and Glen C. Griffin (Fisher Books 1997).

Feeling Good Is Good for You: How Pleasure Can Boost Your Immune System and Lengthen Your Life by Carl J. Charnetski and Francis X. Brennan (Rodale 2001).

Longevity: Reverse the Aging Process and Stay Young with Clinically Proven Alternative Therapies by W. Lee Cowden, Ferre Akbarpour, Russ Dicarlo, and Burton Goldberg (Alternative Medicine.com, Inc. 2001).

The New Millennium Diet Revolution by Keith De Orio, M.D., with Robert Dursi, C.N.M. (Prominence Publishers 2000).

The Mediterranean Heart Diet: How It Works and How to Reap the Health Benefits, with Recipes to Get You Started by Helen V. Fisher and Cynthia Thompson (Fisher Books 2001).

Turn Up the Heat: Unlock the Fat-Burning Power of Your Metabolism by Philip L. Goglia (Viking 2002).

Growing Yourself Back Up: Understanding Emotional Regression by John Lee (Three Rivers Press 2001).

Unleasing the Warrior Within: Using the Seven Principles of Combat to Achieve Your Goals by Richard Machowicz (Hyperion 2000).

Dr. Murray's Total Body Tune-Up by Michael T. Murray (Bantam 2000).

Fight Fat After Forty by Pamela Peeke, M.D., M.P.H. (Viking Press 2000).

Lose Your Love Handles: A 3-Step Program to Streamline Your Waist in 30 Days
by Mackie Shilstone (Perigee 2001).

A Roadmap to the Soul: A Practical Guide to Love, Compassion, and Inner Peace
by Holly Kem Sunseri and F. Dean Sunseri (TVW Publishing 1999).

*Why Meditate? The Essential Book About How Meditation Can Enrich Your
Life* edited by Clint Willis (Marlowe and Company 2001).

*The High Performance Mind: Mastering Brainwaves for Insight, Healing, and
Creativity* by Anna Wise (Tarcher Putnam 1995).

The Glucose Revolution: The Authoritative Guide to the Glycemic Index by
Thomas M. S. Wolever, Jennie Brand-Miller, Kaye Foster-Powell, and
Stephen Colagiuri (Marlowe and Co. 1999).

Additional Resources Online

www.eatright.org

www.turnuptheheat.com

www.pfcnutrition.com

Center for Anxiety and Stress Treatment: www.stressrelease.com

Health Net: www.healthnet.com

The Institute for Stress Management: www.hyperstress.com

My personal Web page: www.mackieshilstone.com

Omega Institute for Holistic Studies: www.omega-inst.org

Ochsner Clinic and Hospital: www.ochsner.org

Dr. Carl Lavie's Web site: www.myheartrisk.com

Information on Soy Products: www.revivalsoy.com

Yoga Journal: www.yogajournal.com

*on*health: www.onhealth.com

Web site for Dr. Dean Sunseri and Dr. Holly Kem Sunseri:
www.Ihaveavoice.com

Leadership Training, and Seminars: www.coachu.com

Medical Information and Resources: www.WebMD.com

Estimate Life Expectancy: www.livingto100.com

Index